Other Books by Allen R. Remaley

The Hunter Model and Its Application to Teaching Foreign Languages

A Hint of Jasmine and Lavender: An Erotic Romance

Susquehanna Odyssey

The Teacher's Playbook: A Guide to Success in the Classroom

In the Shadow of Allah

The Awakening of Annie Hill

Letters Late: Things Left Unsaid

Midnight Lullaby: A Tender Tribute to a Woman

Muhammadville

Reflections of a Disgruntled American Gargoyle

The Magician

Ya Should'a Been There

The Tree Climber

"19'

The Dream Catcher

The Marilyn Chronicles: One Man's Effort to Become a More-Understanding Dementia Care Giver for his Wife

DR. ALLEN R. REMALEY

authorHOUSE

AuthorHouse™
1663 Liberty Drive
Bloomington, IN 47403
www.authorhouse.com
Phone: 833-262-8899

Published by AuthorHouse 01/26/2023

ISBN: 978-1-7283-7894-7 (sc)
ISBN: 978-1-7283-7893-0 (e)

Print information available on the last page.

Any people depicted in stock imagery provided by Getty Images are models, and such images are being used for illustrative purposes only.
Certain stock imagery © Getty Images.

This book is printed on acid-free paper.

Dedication
To Marilyn

CONTENTS

PROLOGUE

If you have been told, and if you believe that there is no cure for Alzheimer's and its lethal relative, dementia, you are correct. If you have encountered either of the variations of the above and are not dismayed by the challenge they present, then you may join my team and win the battle. In short, it, the game plan for an attack and a win over these insidious diseases is simple: meet it head on, smile at its ugliness and the person you care for, as well as yourself, will walk proudly to victory.

Five years ago, my spouse, the love of my life, was backing our car out of our garage. In the process, she sideswiped our pergola, put a slight dent in the car and scraped paint off the still-sturdy pergola. No big thing. Dents can be pulled out, and paint covers such mishaps. However, there were other signs which led me to believe that my wife should be checked out by a neurologist.

My admiration for a person who deals with the nervous system of human beings, a neurologist, leaves me in awe. That person has completed four years of undergraduate school and another four years of medical school. After graduation with a medical degree, four more years of internship, a period of further learning, such scientists move on and practice their profession. Alzheimer's and dementia are just part of the many human deficiencies these people confront. But these last two, these diseases considered to be without cure, concern today's adult population, and they cause disdain, confusion and depression for those who provide care for those inflicted with the diseases.

Before our initial meeting with our neurologist, my knowledge of dementia was like beginning the study of a second language. The sounds, vocabulary and transformational grammar of the disease was mind boggling. At our first meeting with the doctor, my wife was given an oral and written test. As she sat for the exam, she was given questions and asked to perform mental acuity proofs. "What is your date of birth?" "What day of the month is this?" "What is the total of 2022 minus 1959?" The answer to that last question is 63, the number of years my wife and I have been married. Then came the space/distance test. My wife was asked to draw a clock, something she had not been asked to do since grade school. Her rendition of a clock was something which resembled Salvador Dali's 'Melting Clocks'. A few other tasks were performed, and finally, my wife of 63 years was diagnosed with a late-onset of dementia.

So what?! We were both in pretty good shape physically. We played pickle ball five times a week. My wife walked almost daily a couple of miles. She was having her hair done on a regular basis, and her nails and their color was always chip free. Now, let's get this straight!

As an adult male, I do not understand a lot of things, but I do know that hair and nails to a woman seem to be like body armor in the middle of Chicago; you don't leave home without it. Shortly after our first visit to our first neurologist, Madame stopped cooking meals. After all, she had done that chore for many years, and taking on that task made me think of myself as a French chef. Now, after four or five years, my bouillabaisse is as good as anything I ever had in Marseille, my paella is as good as any you might find in Madrid, and my Southwest chili is smokin'. In short, the task of coming up with meal preparation had been solved, and an unnecessary weight taken off my wife's shoulders. Ah, but I wanted to know more about what my wife and I were going to encounter.

ONE

The Support Group Meeting

In the fall of 2022, one of my former Marine friends suggested that my wife and I join the Saratoga Springs, NY, Senior Center. We both fit the age criteria, and it proved to be an interesting place to frequent in the weeks to come. Classes such as Spanish, chess, card playing enabled me to enhance my foreign-language skills, and I was made aware of a session on 'Understanding and Responding to Dementia-Related Behavior', a presentation sponsored by the Alzheimer's Association. Knowing that such things might make me more able to cope with the disease and its consequences, I joined the session directed by a representative of the above association.

A brief overview of how to intervene effectively in this training program for non-professional caregivers was conducted. We learned that experts suggest that more than 6 million Americans age 65 and older may have Alzheimer's. Many more under the age of 65 also have the disease. We were told that unless the disease can be effectively treated and/or prevented, the number of people with it will increase significantly if current population trends continue. This is because increasing age is the most important known risk factor for Alzheimer's and its tag-a-long neighbor---dementia. It was explained that people with the above diseases have trouble doing everyday things like driving a car, cooking a meal or paying bills. The infected person may ask the same questions over and over, get lost easily, lose things or put them in odd places, and find even simple things confusing. Some people become worried, angry, or violent. With the exception of these last three symptoms, my wife fit all of the above categories.

At the end of the overview, the session was open to those in the audience, twelve women and one man…me. Attendees were asked to state their situations. That was a mistake. For twenty minutes, every woman in attendance vented. Some caregivers complained that their patient was belligerent, unwilling to cooperate and nasty. Some of the responders seemed to be proud of the fact that they were in control like some prison warden, and they viewed their situation as one of empowerment; they would control the person for whom they were giving care. What they offered in the way of the dilemma they were facing was so depressing, so intolerant and so negative, that, at one point, I had decided to leave the meeting and silently go home. But I stayed, and at a point at the prescribed end of the meeting, I raised my hand and said, "Please excuse me, but something else needs to be stated."

I began by using some active participation tactics. I asked those present to raise their hand if they had any knowledge of Uvalda, Texas. Some hands went up. I asked them to tell the person next to them what first came to mind. After a very short sharing of information, I said, "Most of you are correct; a shooting by a teenager killed nineteen elementary school children and two teachers. But you know what else happened? Men and, yes, women in blue, ran from that scene and it took over an hour before the shooter was safely apprehended. He, the teenage shooter, was recently tried and convicted and will probably spend the rest of his life in prison. I want to offer you something which has been working for me and the person to whom I give care."

My part of the venting took a slightly different turn. I told my fellow care givers that I had been trained early in my life during my enlistment as a United States Marine, that, in the case of shots fired, we would 'run-to-the-gun', i.e., we would confront the threat swiftly in direct confrontation. There was never any need to ask permission to silence and destroy the opponent, and unlike Uvalde police officers, we waited not one second before we responded with lethal force. We ran to the gun. I explained that this is exactly what I am doing as a care giver. I do not fear the job of being a care giver, and as my brothers and sisters were taught in the Corps, we would win. And, I then went on to explain how my battle plan would work.

TWO

Buy One, Get One Free

While still seated at our open session, I asked how many of those present made daily trips to the supermarket. Hands shot up, heads nodded, and some people said, "I'm there every day." I interjected, "Me, too." But I added that this buy one, get one free logo was a warning. An example was given when I first confronted the disease in my home. My listeners were told that I sometimes asked my wife for help while I was setting up a snack, working on a house cleaning deal or making improvements to things that needed mending. On one occasion, I had asked my wife to turn the heat down on the fireplace and set knives and forks on our downstairs bar…two separate things. The first thing my wife did was turn off the lights to the bar area. She then stopped and looked to me for further direction. I had made the terrible mistake of seeking more than one thing from the person for whom I was caring. Now, understand this: the mistake of asking too much was mine. There was no reason whatsoever to scold, malign or reprimand the woman I loved. That would have been upsetting to both people. Instead, I said, "You know, hon, I like it with the lights turned down low. Thank you. Could you turn the fireplace off. It's getting a little warm."

My wife has become the most-willing person when we have projects around the home, and she likes to feel that she is contributing. Knowing that, I make it a point to include her in almost everything we do at home, and I certainly do not encumber her with more than one request at a time. When and if she follows through successfully,

I make sure that a sincere and positive reinforcement comment is made in reference to her help. Positive reinforcement is such a powerful tool for the care giver, and it beats saying, "I don't need that. Give me the..."

Providing an opportunity for success for the person you are caring for adds strength to both patient and care giver. Grocery shopping gives me many opportunities for positive reinforcement. I make sure that my wife and I both do that outing together. Automatically, as soon as we get out of our automobile, my wife gets our plastic-shopping bag and carries it into the store with her. I sometimes say, "Thank you for remembering the bag. I sometimes forget it and have to go back to the car." Once inside the market, with my trusty shopping list in hand (let's get serious, we need a reminder, too.), we go about filling our cart. I always ask what my wife thinks we need, and she sometimes responds with unbelievable ease, "Do we need cottage cheese?" I make an appreciative response. At the end of our shopping, I again thank my wife for her help and company.

We have made a practice of greeting those we meet on the streets, at places of business and certainly at the check-out counters at grocery stores with a smile and sincere thanks for their service. We both have learned to look at a checkout-person's face as we put our selected items down on the checkout belt. If that person has been having a bad day, has a frown on his or her face, we always say, "Good morning" or "Good afternoon. How are you today?" Almost always, a light goes on and bathes that person's face with a smile. That sense of appreciation is reflected in both the giver and the receiver, and that again, is part of the positive approach to the life we live. Feeling good about others is a trait my wife has developed, and seeing her smile lifts my spirits as well.

The Alzheimer's Association tells us that social connections and relationships affect our physical, mental and emotional health. Research has shown that the single most important predictor of human happiness and long life is having strong social connections. Health-related measures like blood pressure and heart rate improve even with short positive social interactions. My wife and I will continue to use even the supermarket for our laboratory.

THREE

A Healthy Diet and Happy Hour

It has already been alluded to that meal preparation is my responsibility and has been for the last four years. I welcome the job. I am not yet 'Cordon Blue' qualified, but I do pretty well in the kitchen. Fish has been a solid choice for an evening or weekend meal, and I have learned that a nice cod filet can be cut up into chunks, and when cooked in a primavera sauce or vodka sauce, our dinners at home are savored. From week to week, we vary with a mid-morning salad of greens such as spinach, romaine, collard greens, peppers and onions. The following week, I combine an English muffin with cooked egg, cheese, and a chicken or turkey Dagwood sandwich. The entire concoction is microwaved and served hot. As stated above, my chili is super, my Canadian green-pea soup, again loaded with carrots, onions and celery is super. My appreciative dinner partner has never once complained. Oh, yes, there is often a sweet something or other which tops off our selection of cuisine. Variation seems to be working well. Did I mention red meat? For some reason, such a thing does not usually end up on our table. Every once in a while, a do a great ham burg, tomato, lettuce and cheese sandwich… without the bun. And, there is also something else which takes place every day---happy hour.

'Wait a minute, Allen, you do not have alcohol at those sessions, do you?' Are you nuts? Of course, I do? But Madame et moi only do happy hours on days which end in 'd,a,y'. My wife has a half-glass of a good French Sauvignon Blanc. I do a very cheap version of a California red, and I do not limit myself to a half a glass. Nothing more needs to be said here. However, at happy hour, a good music station from a mini-Google machine adds to the atmosphere. My wife and I discuss what we accomplished during the day. Every so often, more so now that a diagnosis has taken place, our next-door daughter drops by and we all celebrate the day together. That takes place only in Upstate New York where we live. Arizona is another story.

May through November is spent in the Northeast. December through April is spent in Scottsdale, Arizona where we have a small two-bedroom, two-bath condo in a gated community. Our condo is located in a three-story building, and we are located on the ground floor of that building, and our patio looks out upon a small walkway and thoroughfare. Passersby and say hello as my wife and I are enjoying a happy hour together, and it was in such encounters and greetings that we started encouraging residents to join us inside our building at a large-room gathering place. That started an almost every-day get together with others, and that socialization was healthy for all of us. Very soon, holidays and special events were celebrated, and Friday night and weekends were set aside for birthdays, and the sharing of gourmet offerings. That lifestyle activity combined with daily pickle ball outings contributed to a life-extension for both my wife and I.

The above activity takes place in a room called the Belliagio Room, and our building, one of several has gained a reputation as the most-social area in the entire complex. The other buildings' residents are not blessed with a sizeable area for such socialization, and some jealousy does rise its head every so often. However, the goings on at our building is a story for another time.

FOUR

Brad Pitt and a Backward Progression

Dr. Allen R. Remaley

Progressing backward? Is such a thing possible. The wording of such a thing would seem to be incongruous. But it is not in this case. In 2008, Brad Pitt stared in a film entitled, 'The Curious Case of Benjamin Button.' In that film, the actor is seen to transform from an octogenarian to middle age, to a young war-time hero and finally to the moment of his birth. The strange thing about this story, as far as my research has disclosed, is that no one, neither a neurologist, social scientist, nor a movie critic has ever mentioned that just maybe, the story portrayed someone suffering from dementia. The symptoms of such a person are similar, i.e., short-term memory is fleeting, but the past becomes more important than the immediate present. My wife's present state reflects such a thing.

Marilyn's short-term memory is momentary. A question seemingly understood must be repeated. A task, once easily completed, is now a struggle while she mentally searches for the solution. Asking for some small thing, the selection of a tea cup, spoon, table setting fixture, or other item related to the moment will produce the most unlikely offerings. If help is asked in finding the proper cooking tool, only one thing at a time must be verbalized, and the item produced might not have anything to do with the solution to the problem---the thing asked for. But that is no reason to be disturbed. Marilyn has other strong things to offer; she can conjure up the past with her remembrance of things, and as she slides backward in time, a certain newness is offered up for view.

At the present time, my wife has slipped backward in time to what might be described as a renewed adolescence. A playfulness has come about which would remind the onlooker of a pre-teenager. A little fist bump when she encounters me, her husband. A gentle nudge of the elbow in passing from room to room, and such things seem to be part of an appreciated change of behavior. Marilyn is quick to laugh at my weakly-put together stories, and that laughter is like a balm to my soul. So, I use that as my ammunition in this onslaught toward the enemy; dementia hates laughter. And, I never run out of ammunition because even though my jokes are sometimes repeated, they are new to Marilyn.

A backward progression is not cause for concern. It is good to pick out pleasant things from the past. The recording of such things usually have to do with happier times, and that might be part of the brain's defense mechanism in an effort to avoid fear and dread. And, I have discovered something else about the past. Familiarity with memorable things is positive, and Marilyn's recent discovery of my books has brought smiles to her face.

I am by no means a New Times Award-Winning Author. However, I have published thirteen novels most of which are autobiographical. Marilyn is in some of them under the name of a protagonist or special character. Lately, my wife has discovered that reading some of these tomes does light up the past. At times, she will say, "I just read about your finding an old banjo in your grandmother's attic." Or, she might say, "I remember your doing that." Then, I will take that moment and we will iron out its wrinkles that have taken place over time, and we enjoy the past…which is where she is heading. Just this morning, Marilyn was reading one of my books, "Letters Late: Things Left Unsaid." That book contains my thoughts addressed to the deceased, those who died before I had a chance to tell them how much they meant to me. As she was reading, Marilyn said, "I just read what you wrote to our daughter's mother-in-law. That was nice." In fact, I had forgotten that this woman, a person who died too early, was in the book. But for Marilyn, the image brought back good times and defeated a lapse in memory.

I am going along for the ride with Marilyn, and I intend to make it a comfortable trip. To do anything else would be a waste of…time. Thank you, Mr. Button.

FIVE

Television Ads, Candy and Other Medications

At home, our television watching is limited to local morning news programs, documentaries and a few movies. We avoid the very biased evening news channels. Yes, even Fox, CNN, MSNBC, ABC, etc. The anchors of each of those news programs do not read the news, they opine as to what they believe. I am not interested in their opinion. But each of those news broadcasts have many commercials, and a lot of them offer advice as to how to increase cognitive powers. I am amazed that some of the paid programmers, those who actually tried the memory pills, offer up amazing stories about the way they can now see more clearly the world about them. Actor-portrayed spokespersons go on and on about the miraculous awakening which takes place after one or two weeks of taking the over-the-counter drugs. It surprises me that none of these witnesses has ever designed a rocket to Mars. One female drug taker actually proclaimed to understand her surroundings and make sense of everything she encountered. Makes you want to try what they are selling.

In one of our first visits to a neurologist, in my naivete, I asked, "Doctor, what is your opinion of things like Prevagen, Neuriva and Noobroo, the so-called brain supplements?" The neurologist hesitated, and then he said, "Do you like candy? That is what most of it is." In my own research, I found that the advertised supplements were not only expensive, they were not sugar free, and they contained lactose. None of these products were good for your wallet, nor were they healthy supplements. As stated above, I will stick to well-prepared and well-balanced meals. Fruit, vegetables, fish, whole grains and white meats. OK, maybe a well-prepared ham burg without the bread. But there are some prescription medicines one should try.

Our neurologists have prescribed two drugs which supposedly slow the symptoms of mild to moderate dementia. My wife takes both Memantine HCL 5 mg and Donepezil HCI 10 mg in the hope that the progression of the disease is slowed. It is too early to tell whether the drugs work. Twice-yearly visits to our neurologists will perhaps tell us more. There is always an effort by most neurologists to schedule the patient into a trial program. In such a program, one half of the participants receive a trial drug. The other half of the select group receives a placebo. After a lengthy trial run, usually a year or more, findings are reported…good or bad. Participants in those programs receive a small allowance for travel, and most are required bi-weekly visits to the medical office for exams and testing. Such a procedure is time consuming, and it does involve travel to and from the testing stations. As of this date, we do not want to be on the placebo side of the fence.

It must be remembered that, in the beginning of this writing, Alzheimer's and its tag-a-log dementia are both considered to be without cure. As for me, I will remain convinced that fighting the disease head on, i.e., not becoming discouraged, and working together daily for both mental and physical health, is still the best medicine. Dementia must hate us. One of our Marine slogans is this: The Devil says, "You will not survive the storm!" A young Marine says to the Devil, "I am the storm!" And, my storm is not a warm wind blowin'.

Toby Keith and 'I love this Bar'

The dangers of social media have already been discussed. The Alzheimer's Association tells us that while technology can improve social connectiveness in some cases, research finds that those who use social media the most are at a higher risk for depression. It is my opinion that watching the nightly news on big networks can be just as dangerous. At least one other thing mentioned by the association was listening to music. Before anything else is written, my wife and I do not listen to rap. But we do make an effort to listen to many types of the genre.

We purchased a Mini Google sound system and installed it in our downstairs bar area. We enjoy some good French renditions of Edith Piaf, Jacques Brel and others. Some Mexican salsa is played, but for the most part, it is country/western which seems to draw our attention. In Arizona as in our New York home, a bar is part of the furniture, and we have enough stools for a social gathering. However, COVID's intrusion had limited guests at both places, but Madame et moi still get together around 5 P.M. at our bar area. Timing is not that important because we know that 'it is 5 o'clock somewhere'.

Once established at our bar, light hors-d-oeuvres are served, and we enjoy a glass of a nice cheap wine and we discuss the day's achievements. Toby Keith sometimes joins us via the Mini Google, and he reminds us that his bar has 'winners, it has losers, chain smokers and boozers'…No one has ever smoked in either of our homes, but like Toby, we love our bars. It is an area where my wife and I are able to review the day, discuss the good things that are taking place in our lives and relax without ever having to drive anywhere at the end of the evening. Yes, we do have visitors and guests, and it is that socialization which strengthens our claim to mental health.

In Arizona, our bar is on our patio looking out onto a walkway, and as previously stated, we always cordially greet passes by, offer dog bones to their pets (everyone has at least one dog these days). Every so often, these passers-by accept an invitation to join us, and we have had to add six or seven stools to our patio area. When our crowd of friends become too large, we go inside our building to a large meeting room where, over the years, attendees have purchased or have donated card tables and chairs. At times, our get togethers number close to thirty people. So, we are following the Alzheimer's guidelines; we are forming new social connections, and that effort has proved positive. My wife loves other people, and she fits in as though nothing bothered her, not even her dementia. Thank you, Toby.

Will such shenanigans continue? Darn right! It is part of my direct confrontation with the disease. Seeing my wife smile and interact with others is like a warm wind blowing, and it strengthens my will to fight this terrible thing. Can't wait to get to Arizona.

SEVEN

Shrapnel and the Taking of Pills

If you are over 65, have developed the habit of seeing your local health-care physicians, you have probably set up a container for the pills you are required to take. Ours, both for Marilyn and I, resemble an ammunition box for machine gun shells. As we get older, the contents of these every-day items grows, and we are put on a regular schedule as to when these daily doses should take place. Our special time of the day for ingesting these life-extending drugs is after happy hour and before we retire before bedtime. And, it has become a ritual. We would sit opposite each other, and I would confirm such things as date, day and procedure to take our pills. Hers first, then mine.

Over a year ago, Marilyn had exhibited a physical impairment when taking her pills with water, the suggested supplement when swallowing what had been prescribed. She would place the nickel-sized lozenge in her mouth, take a sip of water and cough, choke and spew the thing back at me. The thing ejected would wiz past my ear and ricochet off a window or one of the neon lights behind me (after all, it is a bar). In fear of losing an eye, I knew that something other than water should be used to induce swallowing the pills. So, I decided that pill taking could be not only fun, it could be a nice ending of the day.

Ice cream! Even the word evokes a certain something, a pleasure, and taste buds seem to come alive when that sweet, frozen item is seen, mentioned or offered. However, it, that sweet stuff, is usually laden with sugar. We decided that we would try yogurt instead of water. Better yet, it was agreed upon that fruit-flavored yogurt would be tried. It was time to experiment.

Marilyn's pills were laid out on top of our bar, and the size and quantity of the things laid out reminded me of a game of dominoes. Our container of yogurt was opened, I picked up a plastic spoon, dipped it into the delicious mixture and said to Marilyn, "Big one!"

Marilyn would pick up one of the biggest pills, and upon my direction, she would place it in the spoon containing the yogurt. She would then swallow the entire concoction. I ducked. But there was no return fire. The pill went down without any gurgling, gulping or coughing. Success! The rest of the required pills disappeared one after the other, and pill taking became a looked-forward-to evening event. Not only that, I would not have to make regular visits to my ophthalmologist.

Now, the lesson in all this is simple. Taking care of someone you love can and should be enjoyable. There should be no stigma in helping someone overcome a slight difficulty. On a regular basis, my choice of the pill supplement changes from strawberry, blueberry, peach and other fruits. Like that box of chocolates, Marilyn never knows what she is going to get.

We have met the enemy's effort to make our path through this difficult period, and we have won another battle. Hou-Rah!

EIGHT

Morning Rituals

At the moment of this reading, stop. Do you, the reader, know the exact time, the exact date and month you are in? No, you don't. You had to take time away from your reading and reflect. Sure, all this was done within seconds. For a person suffering from dementia, those seconds become roadblocks and cloud the moment's importance. In an effort to make more sense of the day, time and place of things, I decided that Marilyn and I would sit down and contemplate our day together.

The first thing which takes place in the morning has to do with my lightly knocking on Marilyn's bedroom door and giving her a hug and good wishes for that early hour. A year or so ago, we bought an electric-manipulated bed, one which allows for a slight elevation of the mattress which is better for good back support and keeps the user from rolling on one's side, a procedure which prevents neck and shoulder pain. Good sleep is essential for everyone, and I made sure that Marilyn's bed allowed such a thing. As for myself, I have not slept in a bed for over fifteen years. I use an electric recliner, and that, too, was one of the best things I ever did. Both of us get better rest which is essential to good health.

The next step in our day has to do with coffee. Our coffee pot is set up in the basement area in front of our big-screen T.V. I make the coffee, wait for it to perk, and we have our coffee together and watch the local morning news and weather report. We do not set any time limit for this coffee break, and we sometimes discuss what has just been shown on T.V. But what takes place next is a helpful exercise for both care giver and sufferer from dementia.

In our home, we have converted an upstairs bedroom into an office. Two large desks face each other. Marilyn sits at one, and I sit at the other facing her. With pen and paper, we both write out the day and date of the month at the top of the page, and follow that by documenting the important things of the day such as what we are going to do, why we are going to do that, and what we should accomplish by the end of the day. We set no time limit for that task. At the end of five or ten minutes, I ask Marilyn to read what she has written. Once she has finished her daily log, she reads what she has written. I make an effort to compliment her on her writing, and then I read to her my own prognostication for the day. That little writing lab has made the morning more stable and meaningful, and we both are better off knowing what should be done on that day.

Our writing is followed by daily tasks around the home. Laundry is done. I load the washing machine, put the clean and freshly done clothes in the dryer, and later, Marilyn folds and puts the dried clothes away. We meet certain obligations such as hair appointments, doctors' appointments, pickle ball playing and food preparation. Being prepared and confident about surroundings and time goes a long way in avoiding depression. So, Marilyn and I look forward to every waking hour, and we are still in the fight to make the future ours.

NINE

Trains, Planes and Automobiles

In 1987, Steve Martin worked with John Candy of the film, 'Trains, Planes and Automobiles'. That American comedy had to do with a three-day odyssey of diverted flights, cancellations and other mix ups in an effort to attend a Thanksgiving dinner. Such confusion was, at least to one of the travelers, a source of frustration and anger, something you do not want to encounter if you are caring for a person with dementia. You, too, the caregiver must avoid such mishaps.

My wife and I have traveled thousands of miles when we were younger. Flights to and from Europe, Canada, the Caribbean, the Pacific and other sites in this country and abroad took us to exotic and interesting places. Now that we are older, we are less likely to explore the world. However, for the last twenty years, we have been spending the winter in Arizona, and for us, that trip requires a flight. During the first ten to fifteen years, making the trip from Upstate New York to the Southwest was not difficult. Getting up in time to make the flight, making sure documents needed by airport personnel was taken care of, and attending to luggage and carry-ons seemed to be no problem. My wife was in charge of carrying the tickets and passports. I took care of the luggage. But changes have now been required.

Over a year ago, we landed in Chicago O'Hare Airport for a change of planes. My wife had to use the restrooms, and they were located about a hundred feet from our waiting area. I kept our carry-ons, and she made her way to the restroom. That day, hundreds of people were going back and forth seeking their flights. Restaurants and boutiques were packed with customers, and the movement of people distorted things. After twenty minutes, I began to be concerned. Marilyn had not returned to our gate area. Bags in hand, and in a nervous state, I went to the entrance way of the restrooms. Marilyn was nowhere in sight. Women who had been waiting to use the restrooms had gone in and had come out. No Marilyn. I began to search through the meandering crowd. Some two hundred feet away from the restrooms and headed in the opposite direction was a bewildered Marilyn. Yes, I caught her. I did not scold her, and instead, made light of the fact that she was in a crowded airport. But I had learned a lesson; always be aware of the patient and her whereabouts.

Traveling anywhere is now difficult. Marilyn and I discuss needs and make ourselves aware of the location of base points (special stores, opening, views), and at restrooms, no matter how close to our gate, I wait and attend to the basic needs. I now handle tickets, identification cards, and other needed documents. Doing so makes things less stressful, and important scene-setting condition when traveling with a dementia-burdened person.

Signing up for and getting your TSA verification for boarding is helpful. Going straight to your boarding area without standing to deeply in line with others offers some benefit. Not having to take off shoes, a perk given to us because of age, helps, too. We never fly during the week preceding or following a holiday. People are wonderful, but sometimes, there are too many of them, and airlines are stressed, too. When too many are flying, cancellations occur.

Packing a few snacks in your backpack comes in handy. Cross-country flights are tiresome. Energy is sapped, and the body needs sustenance. Power bars, small enclosed packets of cheese, crackers or rice cakes can be little pick-ups along the way. In spite of the fact that my wife and I enjoy happy hours, we do not do such things when we are over six feet off the ground. That comes later upon successful arrival at our destination.

Now, about those 'automobiles' in the title of this chapter. Being the only driver in our family now, I do not drive cross-country. If I did, it would take me three months, and once at our destination, I would have to start back to my original departure area. *Bon Voyage!*

Spatial Distancing, Games and Exercise

Two years ago, Marilyn took daily three to five-mile walks both in New York State and in Arizona. It was nothing for her to walk our familiar streets, shop and return home bright-eyed and ready for anything. Then, she would tell me that, at times, she would be in quandary as to where she actually was. From time to time, she would tell me that someone, usually a woman, would ask her if she needed help. Both of us knew that from that point on, Marilyn would carry her cell phone wherever she went. Her walks are now shorter, and in Arizona, she remains within the confines of our gated community.

I needed to know more about this new phenomenon, and I looked into concept of spatial recognition, the concept used when you look into a mirror and discern which side of the image correlates with the right side and which with the left. Spatial thinking, a relative of spatial recognition, allows you to understand the location and dimension of objects and how different objects are related. Both these concepts are used in everyday activities including simple tasks like finding the way home from work or deciding what size box is needed for a particular object. These two concepts had been erased from Marilyn's ability to comprehend her surroundings, and both are used in playing games.

Over a year ago, I thought teaching Marilyn to play chess would improve cognition. That was a mistake. Space, time and distance are all part of the game, and I noticed immediately that frustration had set in. We moved on to my trying to improve her playing of pickle ball, a game she had done well at four years ago. However, new techniques and a review of the fundamentals of the game seemed to slip through her grasp like water going through a sieve. It was at that point that I got smarter and realized that although she played pickle ball well, she was not going to enter competitive competition. At that game, she enjoys the camaraderie of people she knows, and when she makes a good shot into the opponents' court, I compliment her as though she had just won a gold medal.

Marilyn no longer walks three to five miles a day, but she does walk to and from her hair appointments, nail appointments, and small shopping trips. She remains in good shape, and at the age of eighty-three, she can beat you at a game of pickle ball. Her physical activity is not limited to walking and ball playing. She helps me around the house, especially when I ask for her input. She handles little chores, and she does them well. But the introduction of something new, especially the playing of chess, will not be on the menu. And, that's OK. New things are not necessarily good for everyone. I would rather see a smile and hear a laugh than see her design a rocket or fly a drone.

ELEVEN

Don't Get Sick!

It has just been reported that the world's human population has reached nine billion. That enormous amount of people is beginning to stress us in so many ways, and it will continue to do so for years to come. Feeding the world's population will become a major problem. We are already depleting the world's oceans of fish, a major food supplement for millions, and in spite of agricultural improvements, our food supply is waning. Remaining in good health is a major concern for care givers. But there is something else which is cause of concern---variants of COVID 19.

The pandemic which began a few years ago is still with us. Yes, we have one vaccine after another. We have flu shots and other preventative inoculations which supposedly will keep us safe. However, impure air, something which might be causing respiratory disease, is now a rising concern. For a care giver, remaining in good health is essential to successful protection of a loved one.

Just recently, major chores around the home (lifting, moving furniture, cleaning) stressed both my shoulders to the point where I had to pay a visit to the hospital's E.R. Marilyn no longer drives, and yes, I could have called a taxi, Uber or asked a neighbor for help. But time was of the essence, and I needed immediate attention because there were things at home that needed to be done. With one arm still functional, I drove myself to the hospital, was diagnosed by a physician and was given pain medicine. Marilyn stuck with me the entire time, but she gave indication of knowing that my being able to function was essential to both of us.

For the better part of a week, my ability to carry on in an efficient way was jeopardized. Little things like laundry, meal preparation, house cleaning, grocery shopping and paying bills began to put stress on me and, of course, the person for whom I was caring. I do know now, that even if a hospital stay would have been recommended, I would have refused to comply with the request. And, do not forget, even though wounded, some of the combatants refuse to leave the battlefield. Not only that, I was having fun. At the moment, I am back on track and able to function above 90% efficiency. But things could have been worse.

Marilyn noticed a difference in my demeanor once the pain medicine took effect. In the evening at happy hour, she would say, "You're looking better today." About the third night after she had repeated my looking better, I asked Marilyn, "Hon, should I inquire about being a male model?" She immediately responded, "Yes, you would be great." I answered, "OK, do you know what I would model?" She said, "No, what?" My answer turned out to be just what the doctor had ordered, and I said, "I am going to model athletic supporters." A burst of laughter from my wife proved that I was back on track.

My advice is this: don't overdo things which, in the past, might have been normal. The refrigerator might not need moving every other day for cleaning. Carrying heavy items around the home is not going to build muscle; after the age of fifty-five, muscle building does not occur. Slow down. If your physician has suggested flu, COVID or other shots, get them. Wash your hands, and if you develop symptoms of something which need attention, do what is necessary. But your remaining in good health is tantamount to the successful care of that person next to you.

In spite of the increase in world population, do the best you can with what you have. Maintain a healthy diet and life style. You will be a happier person. So will that person for whom you care. One last reminder. Every time your plane is about to take off, your flight attendant holds up an example of an oxygen mask and tells you, "If masks fall from the ceiling in case of emergency, and if you are with children, put your mask on first." The reason for that is that the care giver must be ready to do what is necessary for those cared for.

On the day of graduation from Marine Corps boot camp in Parris Island, South Carolina, I felt myself ten-feet tall and bullet proof. I get shorter every year.

TWELVE

Day to Day Transitions and Observations

My layman's suggestions for care giving are certainly not those advocated by the American Alzheimer's Association. The above suggestions are those which fit my own personal and intimate relationship with my wife. The following 800 number will get you more information if you are so interested: 1-800-438-4380. The following documentation concerns happenings, viewings and recognitions that have come to my attention and my way of handling them. This log will perhaps come to the attention of our children, and hopefully, they, my son and daughter, will know that their mother was not abandoned by their father.

11/17/2022: Last evening, we were preparing light offerings for our nightly happy hour. It had been decided that black olives (Black Olives Matter), dusted with parmesan cheese and hot pepper flakes would be good. Some fruit, an apple and a pear would round out our hors-d'oeuvres, and I asked Marilyn to choose one or the other thinking that offering a choice would be good. Seconds turned into a minute before any response took place. I said, "You know, you did mention that our Bartlett pears had tasted good." The choice had been made.

11/18/2022: This morning, on our way downtown to run errands, we arrived in front of my wife's favorite nail salon. She went in, made an appointment and returned to our car. Once seated, she held up her appointment card, slipped into her jacket and said, "Will you remember where I put this?" I looked at her and said, "Put what?" She laughed out loud. Minutes later, we arrived at our local Senior Center in order to get ready for our 11 A.M. Spanish class. We both needed a key-card in order to check in. Marilyn could not find hers, and not knowing the exact word for the key-card pass, she said, "What is it that you have and I don't?" Without thinking, I said, "Brains?" Marilyn's laughter could be heard inside the center, and it saved my embarrassment.

11/19/2022: Yesterday, I dropped off Marilyn at her nail salon where she promptly made an appointment for a new nail color treatment scheduled for today. Moments ago, she came into a room where I was working and said, "Hon, do you remember where I put my card for this morning's appointment?" Now, let us be truthful about such things. First of all, nail appointments like hair appointments and doctor's appointments are important, but they are not life-threatening, and there is no reason why a care giver should be upset about a misplaced appointment card. Knowing this, I tried to be as calm as possible and said, "Yes, yesterday, you asked me to remember where you had placed the card, and I noticed that you had placed it in your jacket pocket. Do you know where that jacket is?" She immediately found the jacket and looked in its pocket, but she did not find the card. New problem!

We then searched where that card might have been placed, and we searched the common areas where things usually end up. After a few minutes, in plain sight on a picture frame on her desk, we found the missing appointment card. We laughed at the mysterious missing card's discovery and agreed that in the future, all such cards would be paper-clipped to Marilyn's appointment calendar…something we had agreed upon in the past. Marilyn was on the verge of crying. I showed her that her appointment card was nothing but paper. I told her that it was not a tiger. All was fine. But the past had moved on. Will such searches occur in the future? I hope so. The search/find game is becoming interesting, and I am developing a Sherlock Holmes-like skill. No big thing folks, and it is nothing to get upset about. Play it forward.

THIRTEEN

Reminiscences of a Frustrated Writer

Recently, I suggested to Marilyn that she read, and she did. During the day, she would pick up a book lying around the house and read it. When asked later to describe what it was that she had read, very little having to do with either the action or the plot of the text was forthcoming. In spite of that oversight, thinking that more familiar topics might be both appealing and familiar, I suggested that Marilyn read some of the books I had written. Over the last fifteen years, I have written and self-published thirteen books. Nobody reads my works, but most of them have an autobiographical flavor, and the action takes place in areas where Marilyn and I have lived, visited on long trips, and studied together. All my books are lined up on her morning writing area, a desk set up opposite mine in our study. She began reading my books for the first time.

One of the first books chosen was 'Letters Late: Things Left Unsaid'. In this book, I had encapsulated my thoughts and addressed them to those whom I had known and who had influenced me to a great degree. All of those letters were addressed to now-deceased persons, and the collection had to do with things that should have been said while these addressees were alive. Marilyn had known all of the people to whom I had written. My grandmother, Marilyn's parents, relatives, fellow Marines, school mates and teachers. As Marilyn began to read, she was swept back fully into the past, and moments forgotten were recalled. As she read, Marilyn had said, "Allen, I never realized that you had written to these people. I remember…" And, that was the key, for a brief moment, faces and stories became familiar.

Marilyn is now on the third of my thirteen books, and during the day, she will often say, "I had no idea that he/she did that. I should have started this a long time ago." But the fact that she has started to become more familiar with a forgotten period in her life is a good sign. Will she be able to relate happenings from those books this evening? Probably not, and that should not be expected. What is important is this: Marilyn feels more closely associated with her life and mine. Could the same thing be done with a photo album? Maybe so. However, the danger of a second person saying, "Do you know who that is?" Anything you do to stimulate the mind's ability to acknowledge the past should not be a test. Such practices frustrates the viewer as well as the inquisitor. How photo albums are handled requires sitting down and writing down a lesson plan.

If I were going to dust off some of our old photo albums, I would make sure that a facial-recognition test was not given. Instead, I would play the role of Rick Steves, the travel writer. During his shows, no questions are asked as familiar and not-so-familiar places are described. If the watcher says, "I remember being there. Isn't that interesting.", then you are on the right track. So is the person to whom you are giving care.

FOURTEEN

Prescription Medicines and Their Importance

Whether it is over-the-counter health supplements or physician-prescribed medicine, there should be some kind of assurance that what had been advised is taken on a regular basis, and that whatever has been suggested is kept in an area known be both the person needing those drugs and certainly by the care giver.

For Marilyn and me, our storage area for such things looks like a fishing-tackle box used by an avid angler. Both of us are octogenarians, and our supplements and drugs are stored in a small refrigerator in separate plastic bags for easy perusal. Whatever may be the case, the items placed in those containers must start with a visit to your general practitioner. At that appointment, ask that the doctor explain to both the patient and to the care giver exactly what the recommended prescriptions will do. Whether or not the description is remembered, most prescriptions come with a readout explaining the drug and complications when taken with other such items. Your local pharmacist will also assist in giving explanations of each drug taken.

As stated above, designate a special place where your prescriptions are stored. Your next step should be an accepted time of the day when your drugs are ingested. For Marilyn and me, end-of-the-day activities include taking our medications. It is easier to choose a time and hour when you take your prescriptions, and a regularity will help in being consistent. You and the person for whom you are caring should not encounter a time when you cannot recall taking what has been prescribed.

In an earlier chapter, it has already been stated that Marilyn is now taking her pills with flavored yogurt, a more pleasant and looked-forward-to method. But before those drugs are administered, it should be confirmed by both parties that the exact number of the prescribed drugs are available. Small, plastic, day-to-day containers work well in keeping required dosages on track. Included in this procedure is the filling of those receptacles. In the beginning of our adventure of regular night-time pill taking, I would watch Marilyn as she diligently filled each day's holding area. She counts out her pills, sometimes too carefully, but I do not intervene unless I notice a discrepancy or a repetition of one pill or another. And, keeping track of what is left in each separate pill container is important. It is not necessary to visit the pharmacy too often; refill requests can be made by phone, but it is the care-giver's responsibility to assure that the required pills are on hand.

Marilyn and I have made pill taking into a happy time. When finished with our ritual of putting the right things into our body, we silently give thanks for having done what was necessary. We do not sing out our accomplishment. But a smile of having achieved the task is all that is needed, and we move on to whatever comes next in the evening…watching re-runs of some now off-the-air shows.

FIFTEEN

Athleticism and Socializing

As stated previously, keeping in good physical condition through exercise and diet is essential to both mental and physical health. Marilyn is a girl born at the end of the Great Depression. She grew up in the clay and coal fields of Western Pennsylvania. In her family, girls did not ride bicycles; boys did. Girls did not wear jeans; boys did, and it was not until she moved to a bigger community and was introduced to girls' physical education classes that any type of exercising was offered. Title IX rules concerning girl's athletic teams had not yet been passed, and it was after our being married that Marilyn was introduced to racquetball. In her late thirties and early forties, she would stop at a court club and play racquetball before coming home late in the evening. She became good at it. But that sport has since become less attractive, and she moved on with my encouragement to something else---pickle ball.

Americans have become fascinated with that sport. Almost every small town and community have hard surfaces devoted to pickle ball, and many tennis players are swiftly becoming converts to the sport. Players of all ages are learning rules about the 'kitchen', the 'dink' and net play, and pickle ball is a sport that Marilyn plays well. Lately, I have made the mistake of trying to improve Marilyn's ability and skill level. However, there is something to be learned here---old dogs and new tricks has come into play. It took me too long to learn that anyone suffering from dementia has difficulty with eye/hand/muscle coordination. At first, I believed that Marilyn was purposely thwarting my efforts to show her how to improve her play on the pickle ball courts. My Christmas tree bulb has a tendency to flicker. Now, however, when Mr. Instructor has something to say, he is silent. In Spanish, the expression, *"Boca cerrada, no entran moscas.";* 'A closed mouth does not trap flies." So, I back off, keep my mouth shut and watch a woman play pickle ball and smile every time she makes a great shot.

Marilyn and I play pickle ball three of more times a week for an hour or two. In the interim, Marilyn walks, something she used to do every day. She used to spend two or more hours walking to her favorite stores. But as one might expect, directions and their locations are not always clear. Lately, there have been times when she became confused as to what street, what stop sign and what direction she should take. On some occasions, a kind passerby would notice a hesitation on Marilyn's part and ask her if she needed help. I love such people. Now, Marilyn's walks are not as far as they used to be, and upon my advice, she never leaves home without her phone. But it is still pickle ball that has captured her imagination.

Some of the people with whom Marilyn plays are aware of her situation. Those kind individuals seem to love the fact that while Marilyn is on the court, she is happy, talkative, and enthused with the camaraderie of others. It is this exercise, this physical effort which has strengthened Marilyn's confidence, and it has allowed her to be just as good at the game as any eighty-year-old could be. She is capturing some of her youth which had been denied her years ago.

On the courts, Marilyn is a delight to watch. The facial expression she makes is candy for my eyes. So, games and exercise are important. I made another mistake a year ago trying to teach Marilyn the game of chess. Big mistake; line arrangement, individual quirks of positioning and rules (new ones) proved to be frustrating. If the person you care for likes playing cards, encourage it. If they like putting together jigsaw puzzles, supply them. If they like reading, write some books. I did. Not everything works. Stick with what does.

SIXTEEN

The Important Things

Dementia is such a thief. It robs a person's dignity, and it is no Robin Hood; it gives nothing to those in need. However, we do have weapons in our fight against this invasive species. Make a list of the things the person under your care needs or wants. Special tastes in food or snacks. However, there seems to be a lessening importance in food preference as time goes on. Make notes for yourself, and be aware of changes. Such changes in tastes might not be of interest or appreciated in discussions. Keep them to yourself. But if you are dealing with a woman who was always aware of how she presented herself to the public, make sure you take into consideration likes and dislikes. For Marilyn, I make every effort to keep track of hair and nail-coloring appointments.

Because I am a binary male, I sometimes lose sight of the importance of such things. But after Marilyn's hair appointment, there is reason to celebrate; her entire demeanor improves. If you or the person for whom you are caring is lucky enough to find the right hair stylist, that is a good thing. Here in Saratoga, Marilyn found such a person, and when I get chance, I compliment that professional, and sometimes, I leave a substantial tip for the work done on Marilyn's hair. And, by the way, my eighty-three-year-old wife still looks good, and I tell her so. Of course, there is at least one other area of good grooming which comes to mind---nail color.

Last week, it was time for a renewal. The color of Marilyn's nails had been almost erased, and we discussed what might be a change in beautifying the nails. The color chosen was burgundy, something she had not ever worn. As it turned out, that color was perfect for Thanksgiving, and it fit perfectly with the color of my Cocobon Dark, the wine I consume at happy hour. I use that reference when we relax in the evening, and I praise her selection of hues. You do not need a vivid imagination for coming up with a word of praise. Both the person in need and the care giver benefit.

Make sure that the compliments offered are sincere. The sufferer from dementia is still able to discern the meaning of a smirk, a smile or a scowl. Do not allow a compliment to become something obsequious. One of my favorite French novelists, Antoine de Saint-Exupery said, "Only the heart can see that which is invisible to the eye."

If the person to whom you are giving care is a binary male named, John, Jack or Bill, I leave you with this thought: it makes no difference. That person is a human being. Ask what needs to be done to preserve his dignity. Take the steps necessary to make his and your pathway less cumbersome. Both parties will feel better about being alive.

SEVENTEEN

A Mnemonic Hold

Very often, especially in the middle of a T.V. soap opera, a review of the past few chapters takes place and reminds the viewer of what has taken place. You, the reader, do not necessarily need such a thing. I do. So, this is my aide-memoire which will serve to keep me focused on what it is that I must do in caring for Marilyn. And, I will begin by reviewing some of the things suggested by the American Alzheimer's Association.

One of the first suggestions by the above association is, 'Don't argue.' The person cared for who sufferers from dementia has difficulty thinking and reasoning. If, for example, the person under your care says, "I am going home to see my mother, and I am going today.", there is no reason to get upset. You might suggest something such as, "What a great idea. We have to plan first and think of what we might take along." Within a few minutes or more, the thought of going somewhere will have dissipated like smoke going up a chimney.

Another suggestion has to do with allowing for independence. With my wife, Marilyn, she has taken on with some degree of pleasure the washing up of pans, dishes and other items used in meal preparation, and she does a super job in that task. Sometimes, a washed out and dried cooking utensil will end up in our freezer. No problem. I love discoveries. Marilyn has taken the responsibility of cleaning the carpet which covers the steps in our home. While attaching the electric cord to the right electrical outlet is sometimes difficult, it gets done by someone who independently does it on her own time.

Safety in the home is a factor. You do not want an injury to your loved one to complicate the care you are giving. Look at loose rugs, items on the floor which could hinder walking, and by all means, eliminate ladders which might have been used for storing canned foods. Devote your time and energy to lightening the burden of slower than usual mental capacity.

Does the person you care for get tired during the day and want to take a nap? Might be a problem. Too much of a good thing could keep your patient awake during the night. If that is the case, the person you are caring for might want to wander around in a darkened home, and that could lead to an accident. If naps seem important, you might want to shorten them with a gentle nudging suggesting a cup of tea, a mid-day snack or listening to light music. But sometimes, not often, when Marilyn has drifted from reading to a short nap, I will play "You Are My Sunshine" on my banjo. There is no maliciousness in this 'wake-up-playing.' Marilyn awakens and she says that she loves my banjo playing. You might need a nap, too. But don't overdo it.

Setting routines might be a good idea. Somewhere above, I might have mentioned the morning ritual Marilyn and I dance to. She has her own room with a wonderful electronic-leveling bed (no direct reclining; that does not allow for good sleep). Marilyn's bed reclines to a 25-30-degree angle which can be adjusted for comfort. I wake her up, give her a morning hug, tell her that we will have coffee downstairs while we watch the morning news. Shortly thereafter, we go upstairs to our office, sit opposite each other and write out what we expect for that day. We read to each other the suggestions we have jotted down, and then, we go on with the rest of the day which involves pill taking, a light happy hour and a good-night's rest.

Now that I have re-capped what it is that I must do, I feel better having taken the time for a recall of things necessary.

EIGHTEEN

Marilyn's Chronicles 11/25/2022

The following inserts have to do with day-to-day observations that, if recorded, might show either progress or the opposite.

A short while ago, Marilyn picked up the mail from the front of our home, brought it inside, and had a question about a bill that she had received. In the past, such things would have been taken care of without bringing them to my attention. The bill had to do with a co-pay for a visit to her cardiologist here in town. She suggested that we drive to the doctor's office, pay the bill and return home without putting it in the return mail. After a perusal of the bill, I called to Marilyn's attention that the bill and its payment had to be sent to another city for payment. No stress nor strain was expressed by Marilyn or her care giver. That would have been a needless waste of time, and a simple explanation was all that was needed.

11/26/2022: On our little cul-de-sac in Saratoga, one of our neighbors, a female octogenarian and invalid, died over a year ago. Marilyn had been a faithful visitor and would run errands for the woman when asked. Marilyn would sometimes sit with the woman, and at times, would be asked to spend more time talking about what was new in our neighborhood. The deceased-woman's home is now being renovated by construction workers, and Marilyn has been reminiscing over conversations she and our neighbor once had. Lately, perhaps because of the activity going on during the renovation of the home, Marilyn has had a habit of relating the same anecdotes relating to our deceased neighbor. I see nothing wrong with such repetitions. My wife's kindness in helping the woman must mean something, and I listen attentively and compliment Marilyn on having lent a hand to someone. And, yes, sometimes, I will call attention to squirrels, birds and other movement outside our windows.

Later this same day, knowing that Marilyn was encouraged mentally by the work going in our deceased-neighbor's home, we used the Internet to explore what the home sold for and discussed, with pleasure its renovation. We will probably recall those conversations later... Little things, observations about the past, should not be overlooked.

As an aside, while checking my e-mail, the Internet provided an e-mail message about a ninety-three-year-old woman who could remember what she had for breakfast fifteen years ago. It had to do with a Korean fermented dish which, the watcher was assured, would allow normalcy for years to come. I did not check the selling price of the concoction. I wonder whether I should contact our neurologist. Na!

11/27/2022: It's just a little thing. It is nothing worth wringing your hands over---the misplaced measuring cup. Ours is a plastic, letter-designated measuring cup. We use it when I am preparing grits, oatmeal or some other thing calling for specific amounts of one ingredient or another. Today, I could not find our plastic cup. Of course, I started my discovery search in its usual storage area--- the bottom of the kitchen sink cabinet where other such items are kept. Not there. My search then took me to the cabinets above the kitchen sink. Not on the kitchen table.

Not near the stove. I was reminded of times I would hide dog bones from our daughter's dog. He was a four-legged tracking machine, and he always found his bones. I could have used him now. Not in the refrigerator freezer section. Not in the cabinet where pots and pans are stored either. Not giving up, I looked in the upper cabinets where cereal is kept. Voila! I am still the mighty hunter/discoverer. No mention to Marilyn was made about where our trusty measuring cup should be kept. I look forward to the next journey. Thanks again, Forest. 'You never know what you are going to get.'

11/27/2022: Next up, a special challenge. On Friday, December 2, Marilyn and I will be headed for the Southwest to spend five months in Arizona. We have done so in the past, but things have changed. I will now be in charge of passports, boarding passes, flight changes, and going through the TSA inspection booths. Rest stops in airport-terminal bathrooms will be considered, too. In the past, Marilyn was able to do some of the paper keeping, etc. I look forward to making the trip with my wife, and I intend to do so without too much worry about whether everything is problem free during the trip. Knowing that I must be up to the challenge is good, and a little things like my wife's dementia will not interfere with our flight. Bring it on!

Two hours later, same day: Our daughter and our granddaughter took Marilyn out for lunch. When she returned home, she came downstairs where I was working, and I asked her how it went. She said, "Oh, it went very well." I then made the mistake of asking where they had gone for lunch. Marilyn's facial expression allowed me to realize that the name of the eating place had escaped her. She did describe what she had eaten. In such cases, the names of restaurants are not important. Marilyn has had lunch and dinner at Maxim's and at the Jules Verne on the Eiffel Tower in Paris. But now, recalling those places is not important either. Short-term memory is not essential if the food and the company is good. At today's outing, Marilyn was with two people who love her. That, at the moment, is all that matters.

11/28/2022: It has become more evident that I must scrutinize more carefully Marilyn's ability to fill her own pill case. I noticed today that she had put too many of one prescription in the container. Too many of one pill is something which I must prevent, and I will be more diligent as we take care of the filling of our required number of each dose. Something else has come to my attention. The old adage, 'If you like what you are doing, it is not a job.' Helping Marilyn, my wife, is not anything close to a burden.

11/28/2022: Phone calls to and for the person for whom you are caring…It happens. This morning, my wife received a phone call from her youngest brother (she has two older siblings). Phone calls from family and close friends are good. That socializing adds confidence and provides an anchor to the past. When Marilyn began talking, I hinted that the volume be turned up; it is important that you follow the conversation without being too obvious because you might want to be informed just as much or more than the person for whom you are caring. Doing so will avoid your asking questions about people's names, what had been said, etc. Instead, you might want to say, "Roger (the caller) sounded good. He must be doing well." Avoid such things as, "What did s/he say about (someone) being ill?" Short-term memory means just that---facts slip away like grains of sand in an hour glass.

11/30/2022: Keeper of the keys and other such items. It has just been discovered that up until several months ago, Marilyn was the keeper of the keys to both our NY and AZ homes, i.e., before, during and after flights from one State to another, Marilyn had been in charge of maintaining control of the keys to both homes. I took care of boarding passes, transportation to and from the airports, etc. Yesterday, when I ask for the keys to our AZ home, Marilyn's facial expression told me that things were changing more quickly than I had expected; dementia sets its own speed. Our departure for AZ for the winter months is to take place Friday, December 2. Instead of panicking, we joined together in a search of the required keys. Several sets of keys, not necessarily the correct keys, were found. I calmly told Marilyn that this was no big concern. Neighbors in our area have a set of keys to our condo. However, I looked up and jotted down the phone number of an AZ locksmith and put that number in my cellphone…just in case. Little things, minute changes in behavior might be required. If you are more proactive than I, plan ahead…or add certain numbers to your cellphone.

NINETEEN

Pre-Flight Readiness

Now, just what might be the problem getting ready for a cross-country trip. I have done it many times, and I have crossed the Pacific three times by boat, and on that boat, among the 2,500 passengers, not one binary female was aboard. Marines know how to pack. You don't have much more that a seabag and the weapon you are assigned. What could go wrong. But things change.

For the first time in our lives, I must make sure that nothing is left behind, and that I will be responsible for two people---my wife and I. Marilyn is still quite capable of taking care of products needed or felt needed by a person of the opposite sex. I wear no jewelry. She does. I pack no special creams and lotions. She does. I am not sure that I will question any of the items she feels necessary. Why would I? I have enough to do.

We have already talked about house keys. That, I hope, has been resolved. Tomorrow, I will use the Internet and make an effort to get boarding passes. Marilyn no longer uses the Internet. Such things as prescriptions must be accounted for. The taking of needed drugs before we leave, and the storing of what will be needed once we arrive at our destination. I will plant Marilyn's little bag of pills in her suitcase before mine will be securely placed in our little suitcases.

We will travel light. Two small suitcases, one for me, one for Marilyn will be checked in for the entire flight. We each have a backpack, and no carryon will encumber us while traveling. Some people who travel on our flights have carry-ons which would hold a small pony. We don't.

In our back packs, we will have writing material, pens, books, eye glasses and a few light snacks. We will not take alcohol during our flight. I will need every bit of mental acuity available on this first-time trial flight. So, this, *Messieurs et dames,* is part of my flight plan. I need it, the flight and its transfers, to go well.

So, in my back pack or in my hand, I will hold passports, I.D. cards, boarding passes. The keys, of course, have been packed away…somewhere. Once inside the terminal, I must encourage both of us to avail ourselves of the restrooms before board. Marilyn first with me waiting at the restroom entrance. She will wait for me just outside my restroom. And I will assure her that not much time will be spent alone.

Once on board the plane, I will make an effort to get us aisle seats; being able to reach restrooms on four-hour plus flints is important. Our airline, Southwest, has no first-class seats, and that makes it important that I act as a forward scout. And, so goes the battle on the run-to-the-gun. I do not intend to lose any battle when it comes to my being the care person for the women I love. I do wish I had the knowledge of those who have gone before me. That is why these words are written down. Oh, for God's sake. My words can be improved upon. Yours, too.

TWENTY

Long-Term Care for Dementia and Alzheimer's Patients

The above title of this chapter was supposed to be the subject of discussion at our Senior Center this morning in Saratoga. That meeting, I just learned, was cancelled. That left me with no knowledge whatsoever about what might be needed in the future. So, like many of you, I used the Internet. This is what I was able to learn.

Eventually, most people with dementia need outside care, i.e., someone other than themselves. Options are available, and they include respite care, adult-care services, assisted living and nursing home care. For my own benefit, I am going to make an effort to better understand each of these options. Let's look at home health services first.

Home health services include personal care such as eating, bathing, dressing, grooming and toileting. Such care takes into consideration meal preparation and household chores (hey, that's what I do), basic nursing care such as help with medication (me, too), wound care and medical equipment. Thank goodness, we (Marilyn and I) do not need the last two mentioned.

Respite care services, or companion care, provides time for a family care giver (me) to take a break. This service provides the patient appropriate supervision and an opportunity for meaningful social interaction. Respite care might be an informal arrangement with family or friends, but these services might also be available through a community-service organization.

Adult care centers offer a geriatric care manager, usually a nurse or a social worker who can provide services to support in-home planning. Such a manager could evaluate home-care needs, recommend or coordinate care services, assist with short or long-term planning and provide support or recommendations for addressing difficult care issues.

Assisted living is a residential program that provides services for people who can live with some degree of independence but requires additional support. Services may include an individual apartment or suite of a shared-living space, meal preparation, housekeeping, medication management and recreational or social programming.

Specialized dementia care is also available and offers 'memory assisted living' situations which include specialized-staff training in memory care, meaningful engagement and activities based on the individual's preferences and strengths. Visual aids are usually present which include signs or pictures. Enhanced safety measures such as secure exits are also present.

The nursing home is another option. These institutions provide round-the-clock supervision and medical care, and some of these homes specialize with care services tailored to the needs of certain individuals. They are similar to continuing care retirement communities which offer different levels of care as time moves on and demands an adjustment.

The above by no means is all that is available to you, the care giver. Should you have difficulty choosing what might be best for your patient, The National Association of Area Agencies on Aging can help you decide what might be best for the person who needs attention. Planning ahead, from the very first moment any signs of memory hesitancy are noticed is essential to your mental health as well as your patient. But there is one area which no one seems to want to take on---money. Be careful. If your patient is part of a legal trust, the aspect of time in that trust must be very clear. Usually, five years after the legalization of the trust has been signed will determine whether you or your patient might benefit from choice of institution or program. I have heard care givers say, "I have spent enough money on him already." I try to avoid such people. If you are caring for someone who means very little to you, look for help. Years ago, my aunt was taken to an assisted-living home in Rochester, NY. I would visit her from time to time, and it was obvious that the care givers in that institution neither liked their job nor the people for whom they were giving service. One day, we received notice that my aunt had fallen and broken her arm…she was in a wheelchair at the time. My advice to the reader, the person who might be a care giver is this: do everything possible to make both you and your patient comfortable and happy. If you have to look back on the path you took, look back with a smile reflecting the right thing.

TWENTY-ONE

The Cross-Country Flight

On the eve of our departure for the Southwest, a harbinger of things to come occurred. At the time, I was on my exercise bike in the downstairs area which contains our laundry room, bedroom and family room. Marilyn approached me holding several Swiffer cleaning sheets. She asked where the long-handled Swiffer broom was. That tool is one of my favorites, and when the cleaning sheets are attached to the broom, it makes a super dust collector. I told my wife that the broom handle was behind the electric dryer, a machine Marilyn has used many times. Instead of going into the laundry room where our washer and dryer are located, she went into a near-by bedroom. She came back out holding the cleaning sheets with a bewildered look on her face. Sensing that a problem had arisen, I repeated the broom-stick's location. Marilyn went into the laundry room and returned with a dry mop and not the Swiffer broom. She repeated the steps and then returned with a different cleaning tool. I was about to get off my exercise bike and show Marilyn where to find the right tool. But instead, I carefully explained what the Swiffer broom looked like. After several tries, Marilyn successfully located her broom and set to work ridding her upstairs bedroom floor of dust.

Whether or not she was tired, had not focused on once familiar machines, was caught up in the process of getting ready for a long trip or was experiencing something more severe is unsure. However, in the hours to come, I must be especially cognizant of changes. They are coming faster and faster at a rate of speed I had not expected. It is late afternoon. A light meal and final packing will take place, and we will get up at 3:30 A.M. for a twelve-hour trip. I must be ready.

Addendum: After a late-afternoon briefing at which we tried to determine what might have brought on a relapse of mental acuity, we remembered that Marilyn had been to the beauty salon for a hair treatment. At that session, chemicals were used to tease color into her hair. Chemicals! Those chemicals caused a brief shutdown of mental acuity in Marilyn. Later this same day, Marilyn's ability to comprehend become more positive. Could chemicals have altered Marilyn's ability to think? Maybe so. The pandemic of 2020 through the present hints of having been a miscalculated chemical mishap. Who knows?

Getting to the Albany International Airport was not problem. Our favorite daughter (we only have one), Janine, lives close to our home, and she is a good driver. After a thirty-mile trip, Marilyn and I arrived at the terminal, checked our bags and made our way to the TSA PRE; if you are chaperoning a dementia patient, you do not need someone in uniform asking questions about your birth. Go through the training, and become certified as a pre-examined flyer. However, one young TSA, looked me in the eye and said, "Sir, you have to remove your shoes." I responded, "Why thank you, young lady. No shoes are coming off today. I am eighty-three years old. But if you thought I was younger, that is a compliment." Marilyn was standing nearby, so I said, "You know, Hon, I must look like I am fifty-years old." In a very lucid response,

Marilyn said, "Marilyn said, "No, you look more like thirty-five." Thank goodness for little moments like that.

The flight from Albany, NY to Chicago, our layover spot, took a little over two hours. Marilyn was relaxed but she looked very tired. She followed me like a shadow as I looked over boarding passes, time schedules and departures for Phoenix. On my advice, restroom calls were made, and I was sure to stand just outside the female entrance, and Marilyn was assured that I would be waiting when she had finished. She then did the same for me, and our backpacks acted as anchors while she waited. Remember, as a care giver, seeing to toiletries is part of the assignment. Before we knew it, we were getting ready to board our second-leg flight for Phoenix.

As we waited for our boarding time, it was not hard to notice the comings and goings of hundreds of passengers. People of all sizes, shaped, forms, dress, religion, nationality and demeanor passed by as if we were observing a living-human zoo. I made a short trip to one of the shops in the concourse and picked up water and a few snacks. It is not good for anyone, let alone a dementia patient, to travel on an empty stomach. It was time to board.

The flight to Phoenix to Chicago was four and one-half hours. That is a grueling period of time to be cramped like sourdines in seats that do not recline more than an inch. Stress started to build up as we sat side by side in an airplane carrying over two hundred passengers. We began to question whether we would ever submit to the stress of a cross-country flight in order to escape winter. As I was writing down my thoughts, the words on my paper were beginning to run together and look like a second language due to the turbulence of the weather outside our cabin.

Sometime later, we landed at Sky Harbor Airport in Phoenix, gathered up our luggage, two small suitcases, contacted our shuttle operator, and we were on our way north to Scottsdale. Thirty minutes later, we were in our little condo and ready to rest up for the next day. I prepared a light meal for Marilyn using canned goods and rice, and we had intentions of discussing whether we would ever again do the cross-country flight to Arizona. While we contemplated this, we had a knock at our door. We opened the door and were greeted by eight of our friends, most of whom were now permanently located in Arizona all of whom said, "Welcome back. Happy hour down the hall in ten minutes. Shortly, Marilyn and I joined our friends in our building's large meeting room, and we socialized the rest of the evening. Socializing, one of the recommendations for all dementia patients, made us rethink our decision to never try long trips again. We will make that decision later. Not now. Too much fun with other people.

Thinking back to the flight we had just completed, I remembered something. When we were still two hours away from Arizona, a tired and somewhat confused lady sitting beside me, my wife, said, "Are we still on this train? Why is it taking so long?" Marilyn had confused the mode of transportation, and I was not going to correct her; in my opinion, if she thinks that she is on the Chattanooga and Santa Fe Limited, I am not going to challenge her.

I am going along for the ride. So, I answered my wife by saying, "Well, up ahead they might be repairing the tracks. They are only made of wood and steel." I then contemplated whether I would continue the little white lie by saying, 'I will go back to the caboose and check with the brakeman.' But there was a long line at the lavatory. No real reason the further confuse the patient.

TWENTY-TWO

First Day Activities

Entering a living area which had been shut up for seven months entails much in the way of getting the place up and running. Turning and filling the refrigerator demands a run or two to the supermarket. Even though a list is made of the required items to restock the living area, multiple trips will be made to both the market and to the pharmacy. Basic cleaning around the home, light bulb and battery replacement takes place, and confirming Internet, phone and television reception takes place. As stated above, we take part in afternoon happy hours with good friends and those who want to know what is going on in our meeting room. Last night was no exception. Our neighbors had given us a blueberry pie as a welcome-back gift, so last night, we set up a table on which I had cut and served pieces of that pie. I used a stainless-steel serving piece of cutlery given to Marilyn by her mother. At the end of the evening, we cleaned up the area and returned to our living space in the building.

The next morning, I made coffee as usual and set aside a banana (supposedly, potassium is good for Marilyn) for my wife. In the process, I happened to empty yesterday's coffee grounds into the waste basket. There, on top of last-night's garbage was the stainless-steel serving knife. Marilyn, in her willingness to contribute to household chores had inadvertently disposed of her mother's cake server. Now, for some people, unfortunately, admonition might have taken place which would have served no purpose. At first, I pondered how to handle the situation. Replacing tableware could be expensive. I retrieved the serving knife, put it in the kitchen sink and waited. Before Marilyn had come out of her bedroom for coffee, I made another decision. I was going to use extinction.

In my training as a teacher, I had a wonderful, nationally-known educator, Madeline Hunter. Dr. Hunter was responsible for coming up with The Essential Elements of Instruction, the fundamentals of good teaching. Among those essential elements was extinction, the art of ignoring the shortcoming if it is not dangerous or is not in any way crucial to understanding. In the hope that the oversight of throwing away a piece of cutlery would go away by itself, I retrieved the serving knife and replaced it back in the waste basket on top of the other discarded things. And, I waited.

When Marilyn joined me for a fresh cup of hot coffee, from my seat on our couch, I handed a soiled paper napkin to my wife and said, "Hon, would you be kind enough to put this in the waste basket?" She obliged, moved to the waste receptacle, opened it and stood looking into the contents. I said nothing, but I watched closely and noticed a facial recognition of slip-up. Without a word, Marilyn retrieved the discarded item, placed it in the sink for washing and joined me for coffee. I made no mention of what I had witnessed. There is never any reason to question anyone with dementia about their actions. Active learning is over. Sometimes, ignoring the situation, using extinction, will save the dignity of both the patient and the care giver. Thank you, Dr. Hunter.

TWENTY-THREE

Making Connections

The dementia patient will have problems making the decision on what goes with what. What seems to be so obvious to those with clear depth and perception connections is sometimes a source of confusion for the dementia challenged. This evening, just before getting ready for bed, I noticed that Marilyn was having a little trouble doing what was necessary for a good-night's sleep. Hesitant to go to her bedroom (my night-time actions require separate sleeping areas), Marilyn usually watched a T.V. program before falling asleep. I noticed that her light was still on in her room, and I decided to check and make sure all was well.

I lightly knocked and then entered her room. Marilyn's T.V. reception had no picture. She had put on her pajamas and not yet in bed. I hugged her and asked if she needed something (hugs are a vital part of our day together). Marilyn pointed to a cellphone re-charging cord attached to an electrical outlet and asked, "What is that?" Marilyn has no trouble recharging her phone in the early hours of the day. But the day had almost run itself out. I explained what the cord did, and she still had not fully understood its purpose. She needed more information. Marilyn's phone was lying on the floor next to the charging wire. I picked up her phone, showed her how the two came together, and she said, "I am terrible…" I assured Marilyn that such connections are sometimes difficult, and that recharging a phone is not necessarily the most important thing in the world.

Marilyn is sleeping now. She is at peace. Tomorrow will be another day, and we will try to play pickle ball, a sport Marilyn seems to enjoy. She gets along well with others who, for the most part, are unaware of Marilyn's challenge in putting one thing together with another. However, on the courts, her paddle seems to connect well with the little plastic ball, and that is a thing of beauty.

The next morning, after coffee and writing our expectations out for the day, we went to the pickle ball courts. Upon entering the playing area, Marilyn was greeted by those we had known with verbal calls of "Marilyn! Welcome back!" Marilyn went on to play several games, and she did well. That brought smiles to my face, and I realized that dementia patients are usually at their mental peak in the early hours of the day. At the end of our play, I took my wife for coffee and a blueberry scone at our favorite stopping-off place before going home. I felt that I had made a good choice sixty-three years ago by asking Marilyn to become my wife. I have nothing to say about my own pickle ball game; I try to state the truth as much as possible.

TWENTY-FOUR

Social Interactions and Immediate Benefits

Dr. Allen R. Remaley

In the 1960's, I was a young graduate student at Canada's prestigious McGill University. I am not sure how I got there, and that feeling prevails now in that I am encountering the unknown---my wife's fight against dementia. At McGill, one of my courses involved the study of French impressionism art and literature. My teacher was Rene Huygue, the then curator of painting in the Louvre. One of the artists studied was Paul Gauguin, and his Tahitian rendition of '*Qui sommes-nous? D'ou venons-nous? Ou allons-nous?*' intrigued me. Why would he entitle a painting, 'Who are we? From where do we come? Where are we going?'? That pretty much sums up where Marilyn and I are right now.

Every so often, my wife has some very lucid moments. In the sanctity of our morning coffee, she gives me the impression that all is well, and I get the feeling that we are happy. As the day progresses, Marilyn's path is altered, and her footsteps are wiped out as would her steps along a sandy beach as the tide swept in. It is then that I feel that my life is reflecting the words of Paul Gauguin. But I do have the memory of those good moments such as the skill Marilyn sometimes displays on the pickle ball court, or when she unnecessarily thanks me for taking her to our favorite bakery-coffee shop. Like many others, I do not know where we are headed, but I am sure of our path being certain; we are not alone.

TWENTY-FIVE

Tommy, the Psychologist

Yesterday, in keeping with my belief that exercise was beneficial for Marilyn, we once again headed out for the pickle ball courts. Getting into position to play requires an early arrival. In recent years, pickle ball has become the fastest-growing sport in the country, and we were ready to play a little after eight A.M. It is imperative that I not play as Marilyn's partner. She becomes so nervous over the fact that she might interfere with our chances of winning, that she sometimes removes herself mentally and physically from the game. I usually move to a court away from where she is playing. But this morning, I took a seat along the sidelines and just observed.

As I sat there on the bench, I noticed a renewed enthusiasm in Marilyn's play. She seemed to be more focused, more intent to use fundamentals she had learned years ago, and that brought a smile to my face. Just about that same moment, a man against whom I had played the previous day arrived on the courts. He came over to where I was sitting, and I greeted him by name saying, "Good morning, Tommy. How are you doing?" Tommy seemed surprised that I knew his name. Me, too. I introduced myself as I took a seat next to me.

As we sat there, I called Tommy's attention to the fact that I was watching my wife's play on the court. I explained that Marilyn was in the late-stage onset of dementia, and that exercise was deemed to be one of the things beneficial to her health. As he watched Marilyn play, he turned to me and said, "I am noticing something about her play. She is fixed on being in the right place for the return of the ball, and she has what I call 'muscle-motor memory'; she's at the right place at the right time." At that point, I answered saying, "Tommy, I get the impression that you know more about dementia than you are letting on." He answered, "I am a psychologist and have worked in that field for forty years." He went on to say that 'familiarity' with certain things is soothing. Being with those she knows such as her husband is calming. He added that if he were to suddenly show up in an area she happened to be in, such things might add to an unneeded nervousness. That same 'familiarity' extends to the pickle ball courts I was told. I thanked Tommy for his input, and we both agreed that we would play one another soon. In our previous games, Tommy did not do well, and I decided that I would go easy on my serve to this new informant… maybe not. Aren't new acquaintances just the best people!

After the morning games, we returned home for breakfast and prepared ourselves for our daily chores. Minutes later, Marilyn came into our little office/ bedroom. She was wearing no clothing from her waist down, and she was almost in tears. She divulged that something new had occurred---incontinence. Made no difference. I was her care giver, and I loved her.

TWENTY-SIX

The Fear of the Unknown

Marilyn's first experience with urinary incontinence was entered into a running Face Book account under my name. Most readers commiserated with me and subtly expressed concern. One of my friends berated me for having disclosed an aspect of an on-going account of my confrontation with a stealth-like malady. That is too bad, because the more one knows about continence and incontinence, the ease of coping with the inconvenience is calming.

About 33 million people in the United States have some form of urinary incontinence of bladder condition concerns. Urinary incontinence is most common in women than in men. In fact, incontinence affects more than twice as many women than men. About 40% if women aged 65 and older have some form of urinary incontinence.

The most common type of incontinence, stress incontinence, happens when an action puts pressure on the bladder causing urine leakage. Coughing, sneezing, jogging or exercise (pickle ball) or even laughing (I do my best to get a snicker out of Marilyn) can and does contribute to urine leakage. Is this a hurdle over which we cannot pass? Nah, nothing is going to stop us from finding humor in getting older.

Yes, of course, all the above will be discussed with our physicians. But right now, all is calm...as it should be. Later this afternoon at happy hour, I will say to Marilyn, "Hon, from now on, I'm going to be careful where I step when I tell you a joke."

TWENTY-SEVEN

Routing Numbers and Rocket Science

Most couples probably have separate bank accounts. It is not uncommon for both spouses to be employed while raising a family. Getting and accumulating stuff, the things others have, seems to be what drives Americans today. Economic, social needs and entertainment sometimes demand separate checking accounts. Marilyn and I fit into that category.

Marilyn likes to make and go to hair and nail appointments. I try not to interfere in such things because I am unable to understand the importance that carries for the female of the species. Marilyn pays for those appointments with her own checks or credit cards. However, such arrangements call for record keeping and instant access. That led to a problem.

In packing for our trip to Arizona, Marilyn misplaced her blank checks and related material. That was my fault, not hers. I should have managed that just as I manage her medications. I didn't. Now comes the unnecessary trauma of trying to get those banking items by using the phone. Once a connection is made, you hear, "What is your routing number on your checks?" "What are the last four numbers of your social security number?" "What is the secret bank code you were given?" "Who wrote 'Lincoln's Gettysburg Address'?"

Now, Marilyn is on the phone with me right beside her. After all, my voice does not sound female-like. Marilyn is becoming stressed, and she hands me the phone. The bank clerk on the other end of the line whose first language is not English says, "Who are you and what is your affiliation with Marilyn?" "What is your Marine Corps I.D. number?" I got that one right. That is when I asked the bank representative to call me later. I knew that I had things to do.

In a call-back, a more sympathetic customer-service person resolved our situation and assured us that blank checks were being sent to our Arizona address. I took Marilyn aside, gave her a big hug and explained that our day was a good one. I emphasized that she had performed well on the pickle ball court, she has done a great job washing up dishes I had used for preparing brunch, and that not having the correct banking information was not fatal. We discussed the fact that not knowing the proper passwords and other trivia was not going to keep us from today's happy hour. All was well.

Ironically, I am now reading Ken Follett's **Code to Zero.** In his book, a man who had been Harvard educated in science wakes up on the sidewalk without any memory of who he was, where he was and how he got there. He does have some reasoning power, and he goes to a library in search of what affects and governs memory. His findings reveal that there are several types of memory. Autobiographical memory records events we have experienced personally. These are labeled with time and place: we generally know not only what happened, but when and where. Marilyn can sometimes recall such things. It is very much like Brad Pitt's character going in a backward progression.

In long-term semantic memory, general knowledge such as the capital of Romania and how to solve quadratic equations comes to mind. Neither Marilyn nor I fit into this category. In short-term memory, we keep a phone number for the few seconds in between looking it up in a phone book and dialing it on our phone. It is soon forgotten very much like passwords, routing numbers on check stubs and where you put your keys. Knowing such things helps me, the care giver, to recognize that I might sometimes block areas which might cause stress. In the future, my reading will not include such things as number theory, polymer engineering nor the principles of rocket science. I'll stick to banjo playing, learning how to play the guitar and finding a place where Marilyn and I can get a burrito.

TWENTY-EIGHT

Long-Range Planning and Short-Term Memory

Over twenty years ago, Marilyn and I invested in a two-bedroom, two-bath condo in Scottsdale, Arizona. Neither of us were ready to put ourselves in position to end our working careers, but that move prompted me to retire from a job I loved---teaching. That decision coincided with the 9/11 attack on our country by religious zealots, and neither of us were in the mood to enjoy life to the fullest. However, once a decision had been made, both Marilyn and I were determined to make the move and be climate chasers, aka snow birds, those people who sought warmer areas to escape the winters in the Northeast. That decision was a good one, and it is, under the present circumstances, (Marilyn's condition) proving to be medically and mentally one of the best moves we ever made.

Our condo is located in a gated community which consists of several high-rise, three-story buildings and low-level casitas. Our little place, the smallest square footage of any other condo, is located on the ground floor of one of the high-rise buildings. In that complex, a large meeting room was available for social gatherings, meetings, or mid-day gaming. Marilyn and I were the first occupants of our building, and we waited for others to join us. And, they did.

Some retired native Arizonians, mid-America dwellers, Canadians and even others like us, escapees from the snow-covered Northeast, began to fill units in our building. Good people. People seeking a life new to them. Marilyn and I made a point of welcoming these newcomers by verbally congratulating them and inviting them to establish a camaraderie of community living. The first thing we did was to take over the community room and start planning get togethers on a regular basis. Happy hours were established, and we held them only on days ending in 'day'. Weekends were special, and pot-luck dinners, birthday celebrations, special events and impromptu walk-ins took place. Everyone was welcomed. Race, color, creed, religion or whether you were binary or non-binary played no role in our acceptance of newcomers to Bella Vista, the name of our community.

On special-event days (Super Bowl, St. Patrick's Day, Valentine's Day, NCAA play-off games) fifteen to twenty residents gathered in our meeting room and bragged about their home back in wherever they lived during the summer. Summers are warm in Arizona, and one-hundred plus degree days are as common as are the hundreds of humming birds flying around our buildings. But building 25, our building, had built a reputation of being one of the most friendly and fun-loving of any of the other high-rises.

Marilyn and I have a little outdoor patio attached to our unit. Our daughter-in-law, a wonderful, beautiful and talented Hispanic, suggested that we buy a small bar, add some barstools and use it as an afternoon refuge area out of the sun. Before long, that bar and ten bar stools were filled with friends from all over the building as well as those who lived in other units throughout the complex. Very often, the overflow of revelers had to move inside our building to the meeting room. All of us worked together, went to garage sales and picked up card tables and folding chairs. Those items were stored in a closet in our meeting room, and we would bring them out for special occasions or on happy hour nights during the week. And, at the point in time, when all of us are showing age and certain afflictions, the camaraderie built up over the years is paying huge dividends.

Last night, 12/10/22, at happy hour, six or seven of us met in our community room (many other climate chasers will arrive for their winter's stay in January), and we shared hors-d'oeuvres and conversation. Our second-floor neighbor, Jerry, a fellow banjo player, set up his chair and played a few licks. Jerry's playing is loud, but in spite of the volume, conversation never ceased. But the most interesting thing is this: fellow participants made sure that Marilyn was totally involved. One of her friends presented her with an early Christmas gift. Two other friends set up and lighted a small Christmas tree. Great spirit was exhibited by all. Something started over twenty years ago is working magic for a woman, my wife, afflicted with memory loss. Let me suggest that such things take place with others who might feel themselves alone. Such outings put smiles on everyone's faces.

It must be remembered that positive social gatherings will not erase short or long-term memory loss. Nothing will; there is no cure for dementia. But a smile is worth much more than a frown.

TWENTY-NINE

The Presumptuous Care Giver

In my effort to be as efficient as possible in my role of care giver, I try to be to be aware of the newest applications of techniques, methods and trends concerning the attention one should give when caring for a spouse afflicted with dementia. That's part of the job. Something caught my eye the other day on the Internet. An exercise had been developed and tested which, according to the person documenting the film advertisement, would add to the upright stability of the dementia-afflicted person or anyone of increased age.

In the film, it was stated that standing on one leg for twenty seconds or more would increase the confidence and stability of any elderly person. It was added that many elderly people have a tendency to shuffle along instead of taking good steps in walking. All sorts of warnings were given about correctly applying the practice and techniques of this sure-fire improvement to one's stability.

The demonstrator of the exercise told his audience that the person practicing the move should first find a firm piece of furniture on which to hold before doing the prescribed moves. A chair, strong table or upright and sturdy pole would suffice. The practitioner was told to stand firmly close to a sturdy hand hold. Then, without holding on to the support, you were to lift one leg behind the other and stand on one leg for twenty seconds before again reaching for the support area. It was stated that some practice should take place, but within a short time, the person training on the new technique would be more stable while walking and not have any fear of walking. How hard could that be?

I asked my wife, the person afflicted with dementia, to watch while I demonstrated the new exercise guaranteed to improve stability. As a firm hand-hold prop, I decided to use my stationary bike, a heavy machine I used daily. As an athlete, I knew that I could demonstrate the procedure so that my wife, Marilyn could improve her stability. I said, 'Now hon, watch this exercise. It will improve your steadiness in walking or in any area where movement is involved." I held firmly onto the handles of my exercise bike, lifted one leg behind me, and let go of the security blanket hand hold. Within three seconds, I was tottering to the left, and I grabbed back onto the bike. But I knew that I could do better. I then lifted the other leg. Two seconds later, I latched onto my support.

I proudly explained that it would take time to master the exercise but not to be dismayed at its difficulty. Marilyn said, "Let me try." I said, "Sure, I'll stand close to you while you try." Marilyn grabbed the bike handles, raised one leg behind her, let go of the bike, and remained on one leg for twenty seconds. Without grabbing back onto the bike handles, she tried the other leg. This time, she stood on one leg without tumbling or grabbing the support bike handles and said, "I walk every day for exercise. That must be why I do this better than you do." My days of watching television ads are over. I refrained from stating anything about the role I was playing as a care giver. But with practice, my steps should improve. I'm setting a goal of five seconds or more.

Fielding and Asking Questions

In baseball as well as in many other sports, being ready to respond and act appropriately is a big part of any game. The shortstop in baseball stands ready to field whatever comes his or her way. The ball's bounce is anticipated, fielded and projected in a designated way. That type of readiness could be applied to the care-giver's response to questions from the dementia patient. With Marilyn, I am finding that I must not be too quick to answer her questions. I must first let her know that I am a willing listener, ready and willing to respond to her inquiry. It doesn't take any more time out of your day to be patient, tolerant and responsive. First, you must grasp the meaning of the verbal probe.

With Marilyn, I use what I call a backward-buildup. In order to make sure I understand what is being asked, I sometimes re-word her question in a way that she, too, remembers why she asked the question. I do that as clearly as possible and wait for a confirmation. That initial approach, cautious but attentive, will not only relieve tension, it will assure the patient that she or he has not been overlooked. It must be remembered that in some people, short-term memory sometimes erases what has just been uttered. And, your responses to the person who asked the question must be well-thought out before delivery.

Amazon, Prime, Fed Ex and other delivery organizations usually e-mail you that something is coming your way. They announce what is coming, and that allows you to anticipate delivery of an item. The same procedure could be used in your responses to the person afflicted with dementia. In my response to Marilyn's questions, I might say, "You know, that is a good question. Let me think. You want to know whether or not we took our medications. Well, yes, we did that earlier, and now we have nothing further to worry about." Your questions to the patient should take the same form. It should be added that once a question has been asked by a dementia patient, that same question will be repeated within minutes; short-term memory erases the verbal inquiry almost immediately.

If I am going to ask Marilyn a question, I must take the time to set the stage; I must make sure she is on board, listening and ready. With most adults and others of every age, listening is not a well-practiced skill. People like to talk. Getting the patient's attention is important. Eye contact, a subtle verbal nudging might be needed. For example, I might say, "Hon, do you have time to hear something for me?" That is followed by the gist of the question, and even then, a slow, deliberate delivery is needed. Sure, such techniques take time. In my case, I am not going anywhere. All I have is time, and, I am being paid; I have Marilyn's attention. Take all this to the ballpark and enjoy a hotdog. You might just hit a homerun.

THIRTY-ONE

Hospital Visits: Sometimes They are Unavoidable

Marilyn and I have always gotten up early. Sleeping in past 7 A.M. seemed like a loss of time, and this morning was no exception. I had already put the coffee on, shaved, and knocked on Marilyn's door by 5:30 A.M. She was awake, but seemed discombobulated. We had coffee, but she complained about being dizzy. We had already scheduled an appointment with a new local physician for February 20, but we were only mid-way through the month of December. On the advice of some friends from Ohio, we got dressed and headed for the ER in Scottsdale. We checked in at 7 A.M., but it was not until 10 o'clock that things started to take place.

It was unexpected that the next chapter of this account would center on a hospital visit for Marilyn. At the moment, 6:30 P.M., she is being kept overnight for observation, and if it is rest that is expected, that is a non sequitur; hospital trainees take blood pressure and draw blood every two hours during the night, and rest is impossible. Sometimes, the hospital is the worse place to be if you are ill.

Marilyn had been fed, and we will be advised tomorrow late morning about what has been found. Marilyn's blood pressure has been high, and the drug, Lisinopril, has been increased in dosage. A cardiologist, a nice, young, oriental-American who could not look neither his patient nor her care giver in the eye, will keep tabs on her heart. We do hope that Marilyn will be released before noon tomorrow.

What does all this mean for the dementia care giver? Simple! Be vigilant. Be ready for anything. This morning, while waiting in the ER bed rooms, Marilyn needed to use the restroom. A paramedic came in and escorted her to the restroom, but he left her there. When finished with her restroom call, she was bewildered as to where her room was. I was called to where she happened to be. The paramedic is not at fault. I am. I should have escorted her to that restroom. I should have taken charge. I didn't. If I had been wiser, Marilyn would have felt more secure, and that, folks, is part of the care giver's job. I am learning more every day. Please don't criticize me too harshly.

THIRTY-TWO

Aftermath

On the morning after Marilyn's admission to the hospital, one of Marilyn's physicians called me from the hospital. I was told that he was very pleased with the results of tests. No serious heart problems came to light. But she would be hooked up to a monitor, and I would be responsible for maintaining battery-operated apparatus which gave the hospital hourly checks. I was told that Marilyn would be released from the hospital later on Friday, December 16. I immediately got dressed and went to the hospital.

As I document this latest occurrence, I am sitting at Marilyn's bedside early Friday morning. She has not yet had her breakfast, and I am going to suggest a heaping pile of pancakes. I would learn later that, along with other complications, Marilyn's appetite had decreased, and that caused me concern. A healthy diet is essential to anyone experiencing illness. To the dementia afflicted, it is more serious; that person is sometimes not able to configure hunger.

A few days ago, I purchased a book written by Teepa Snow, her 'Dementia Caregiver's Guide'. The book does offer some good information, but nothing, not one word, outlines what the care giver does in the hospital while his patient is being probed, examined, scanned and filmed by X rays. Being in a hospital for long durations or even overnight is taxing. Even my stay, eight to ten hours while visiting Marilyn was challenging. However, I am always impressed with the quality of concern and care given by physicians down to the person who delivers the meal. But let me get back to Teepa Snow's book.

Some good ideas were stated in the book. For example, it was suggested that a daily routine be established. Marilyn and I do that. I make the morning coffee which is consumed while we brush up on the local news on T.V. We then go to the kitchen table where we take our prescribed medicines, Marilyn takes hers with yogurt, something I have already mentioned. Mine are taken with water. We then use a blood-pressure machine and record our numbers, and then we take separate areas on the table and write. We record what might have taken place the night before, we sketch out a plan for the day's activities, and we try, as much as possible, to remember what must be done that day. Snow's recommendations did include an attention to the senses. Taste, smell, hearing, sight, touch were discussed, and each of these senses must be observed by the care giver. None of these things can be overlooked if you are on a hospital visit.

Once you find yourself in the hospital with your patient, you must be fully aware of everything. Think of walking through a minefield. Be careful where you step; there are a lot of things taking place. Carts carrying patients to and from the X-ray department are whizzing by in the hallways. Machines of all kind are on wheels in your area. Secretaries armed with health-information, insurance coverage, personal information and every other bit of data are collecting things vital to understanding the hospital patient. If you are the care giver and in need of hearing aids, put them in; you will be answering a lot of questions from hospital staff. Listen to them.

Be serious in your actions around your dementia patient's hospital employees. Most of them are well-intentioned and well-trained. If you are receiving good treatment from physicians, nurses and support personnel, let them know how much they are appreciated. I made a point of telling one young lady, a black-American…no, let me correct that; an American whose father was a Vietnam Marine veteran. She noticed my Marine Corps hoodie I was wearing, and we had great conversation.

We were given a battery-operated heart monitor, and now, my lesson plans include a daily recording of that machine's output. So, my daily work includes writing out lesson plans, something I tried to perfect in the past. Hospital visitations take their toll. If your dementia patient is hospitalized, you, too, are part of the team which is offering help and assistance. Be alert. Each step you take can be crucial.

THIRTY-THREE

When Faced with the Imagined and Battery-Operated Apparatus

Early this morning, Marilyn seemed concerned with finding something. Lights were on in her closet and in her bedroom. When asked what might be the problem, she said, "I cannot find my wallet. I had it yesterday." Yesterday, she was in the hospital and had checked in the day before. We were released from the hospital late yesterday afternoon, and at no time did I notice any wallet. First of all, the care giver should not ask, "Where did you put it?" That started the trauma. Do not add to the confusion. You might want to say, "Can you describe it to me and tell me what was in the wallet?"

The various places where Marilyn places her possessions were scrutinized. Nothing found. I then began to inquire about the contents of the supposed wallet. "What did you have in the wallet?" Marilyn told me that she had her cards and some money. We determined that perhaps she might have had as much as twenty dollars in her wallet which was not a sizeable sum. We discussed the consequences of not finding the thing which was misplaced, and I then asked how important the wallet was. We both agreed that wallets and money can be replaced, and that worry about such things was not worth the time and effort. I then changed the subject and I asked her how she felt about her new pillow. I had purchased a My Pillow from the well-known distributor, and presented it to Marilyn upon her return from the hospital. We never did find the wallet.

The wallet was forgotten. I carry all of Marilyn's I.D.'s. She does have a purse in which she carries some money and credit cards, and that is kept in a designated area she cares about. I used to write my opinions about illegal border crossings, inflation and the cost of gasoline in Face Book. Those things don't interest me anymore. I've got other things to worry about. Remember the mentioning of the battery-operated heart monitor?

Last evening, after being discharged from the hospital, Marilyn wisely decided to take a shower. We later met in the common room of the building in which we live and had a happy-hour welcome home for Marilyn. We were told that taking a shower would not affect the heart monitor. This afternoon, I decided to re-charge both phone attachment and monitor. I had Marilyn remove her top clothing in order for me to remove the heart monitor from her chest. The monitor was not there. When I asked Marilyn where it had gone, as you might expect, she had no answer. Then, after a second, she said, "I think that I threw it in the garbage." Oops.

I found the monitor in the shower soap dish which saved us a considerable amount of money. Both the phone scanner and the heart monitor are now recharging. Later this evening, I will reattach both and be vigilant as to what actions are taken with machine and body. We are to use the heart monitor for two weeks and then return it via Fed Ex. This care giver thinks that two-weeks-time cannot pass fast enough. Every day, the care giver learns something new. I feel like a WWI bi-plane fighter pilot whose head is on a swivel looking for enemy aircraft, and I am out of ammunition.

THIRTY-FOUR

Concepts and Their Importance

The knowledge and recognition of something already in place and what it does is not of tantamount importance to the person afflicted with dementia. There are too many other distractions which erase the importance of the minutiae, and some incidents are worth repeating. Repetition is good for the memory. On the afternoon of Marilyn's release from the hospital, she felt that she needed a shower. She was right. Once finished, she dressed, and we both headed to our community room for a small get together with friends. I gave little thought to the heart monitor which had been attached to Marilyn's chest before leaving the hospital. We had been told that water would do no damage.

The morning after our get together with friends, I decided that it might be time to recharge the phone-like gadget which communicated with Marilyn's heart monitor. Both instruments needed recharging. When I asked Marilyn to sit next to me and show me the on-body monitor, the little gadget had disappeared. I asked Marilyn where it might be. At first, she had no idea where it was. Then, she said, "I think that I threw it into the garbage." Now the heart monitor and its attachments are the property of the hospital, and after two weeks use, all the equipment must be shipped by UPS to the maker at no cost to the user. If not returned, the users must compensate the hospital for loss. No big thing. Several hundred dollars might cover that. But I decided to retrace Marilyn's steps. The little electronic heart monitor was found in the shower's soap dish.

This morning, after our morning rituals (pill taking, heart-pressure readings, other medical needs), we re-attached the heart monitor to Marilyn's chest. We then addressed some Christmas cards, and Marilyn was assigned the job of stamp placer. I did the writing, addressing the envelopes, and she applied what was desired by the USPS. Once she had finished her job, she said, "I am not taking these cards to the post office for mailing. Instead, I will take them to our little area where we pick up our mail. There's a drop box there." Now that, *Messieurs et dames,* is an opportunity to congratulate your patient. A concept had been recognized and addressed. I told Marilyn, "Hon, I would never have thought of that. How did you come up with that?" She replied, "It must be my brain."

THIRTY-FIVE

Planning and Improvisation

None of us, neither the neurologist nor the care giver knows what is in store for anyone faced with the unknown. All one can do is plan for the present and the immediate future. Days ago, if anyone would have said to me, "Allen, have you noticed anything peculiar about Marilyn's actions?", I would have come up with some poor expression bathed in humor. Not anymore. I do know that the sand running through the egg timer seems to be dropping at a faster speed, and there is nothing that allows me to stop time. That being the case, I have decided to mold the future to my liking and make it as pleasant as possible for Marilyn.

I have studied cases concerning others and how they coped with the challenge of being a care giver for a dementia patient. I recently was made aware of the book, 'Pathways to Wellbeing with Dementia'. In the first few pages of that book, the care giver is advised to simplify, choose one thing at a time and focus on that. The care giver is asked to lower expectations; you are not going to teach your dementia patient the game of chess. Instead, have fun. But there are times when I feel like a college freshman arriving on campus for the first time without a clue as to what I should do. Having been in the position before, I am going to bring that beginning student in a fast-step march to making things more interesting for my wife.

In our building, a fellow climate chaser and I sat down and designed a series of activities that our fellow residents might enjoy…Marilyn, too. Our fellow escapees from the winter's wrath will be introduced to monthly get togethers separate from our daily happy hours, and we will invite everyone to join in and have a good time. Let me describe some of the things we have proposed.

On Saturday, December 31, 2022, we will celebrate an early New Year's Eve. That event will take place in Arizona time from 6 P.M. to 8 P.M. 'It's got to be midnight somewhere!' Participants will bring hors-d'oeuvres for 6 to 10 people with a BYOB side-bar. We will sing Bobby Burns' *Auld Lang Syne*, and something tells me that some cheap champagne will enter into the picture. I might even bring my banjo. Maybe not.

Next up is January 20, 2023, which will feature 'Crock-pot Night'. Building residents and outsider fellow climate crashers will set up their favorite crock-pot selections and share recipes with others. After today's World Cup Soccer game between France and Argentina, there will probably be a good Argentinian malbec around.

In February, you already know what is coming. February 12, we will set up a TV in our community room, and host a Super Bowl Party. Favorite team T-shirts, colors and decorations will set the stage. I'm guessing that sauerkraut and hotdogs will be there. We are not much into caviar. The Mexican Modelo Negra will probably be around.

Kazoo Night will take place in February. The week preceding February 26 will be the hand-out of kazoos. One of our building's residents purchased enough of these musical instruments for all who might attend. They will be instructed to practice at home and perfect their skills at this odd-sounding instrument. On February 26, we will host a 'Kazooing with the Stars' event and winners will be selected. I hope someone does not decide to do the Marine Corps Hymn. Chesty Puller would roll over in his grave. Sorry Chesty. I have to do it; John Phillip Souza will not be in attendance.

On March 17, we will celebrate St. Patrick's Day. The wearing of the green will be in vogue, and I do make pretty good corn beef and cabbage. Other attendees will dream up something they prefer.

Our get together for April 1, *'Poisson d'Avril'*, or April Fool's Day, we will celebrate famous people. Participants will have a name tag placed on their back. A famous person's name will be printed on that tag, and the wearer will not be told who's name it is that they are wearing. Before the evening starts, rules will be posted saying that no one is to divulge the name of any person on the tags. They may only answer "Yes" or "No" when questioned by the wearer of the name tag in an effort to discover who they are. Those people are to try to come up with the name of the person on their back's name tag by a certain designated time. I might have Marilyn be the time keeper.

By this time, you, the reader, have an idea of what kind of place this is. If you do not enjoy having fun with others…In the words of Toby Keith, "It's my kind of place. Just walkin' through the front door puts a big smile on my face. Come as you are. No cover charge" …especially for Marilyn.

THIRTY-SIX

Placement, Discovery and Doubt

Recently, some odd things have been happening around our home. Cooking utensils, things used on a daily basis and some of the less-common but needful items come up missing. Over a week ago, I had removed a stainless-steel cooking rack from our microwave oven. Its presence would not allow for a large bowl to be placed on the cooking area. I had laid that rack aside for cleaning. A few days later, that piece of cook ware could not be found anywhere. But I do know where it might have ended up. Marilyn is not used to doing meal preparation. That, among other things, is my job. I was very careful not to accuse Marilyn of misplacing that metal rack. The concept of that piece of metal was insignificant. My bet is that it was discarded when she collected the garbage.

Misplacement of things such as keys is not something to fret over, and by all means, trying to verbally correct such mistakes is futile. The dementia patient has no knowledge of what such things are used for, and function is not part of their reasoning. Little things such as which way a gate swings is like solving a difficult math problem. The care giver must observe and hesitate before trying to correct a misconception. Doing so preserves a certain dignity, and being understanding keeps the care giver strong. It is all too easy to become discouraged and depressed because someone close to you has lost the power of reasoning. Take your time in such cases and have a cup of tea with your dementia patient. It might taste good…to you both.

In the process of acting as a care giver, there will be times when the pragmatic comes into question. The care giver will ask himself whether the day-to-day routine is worth the trouble or whether he or she has the strength and will to continue. Answering oft-repeated questions, maintaining a continuum of service and the inherent knowledge that nothing will alter the course of dementia's dive into oblivion. All that can and does erode the good intentions of many people. There is no sure-fire advice to the person who begins to doubt his or her service. However, there is one thing to keep in mind---the need of the person you are serving.

Many of you, readers who are now focused on these words, have encountered a child or an adult who inadvertently comes across an injured animal. It could be a bird crippled because of some hunter or another animal abandoned for some reason. Very often, the person who finds himself in such a position picks up the wounded animal and seeks out help from others in order to sustain life. You, the care giver, are that person. Turning one's back on a living, breathing entity in need would injure the soul of both invalid and observer. It is much better, I think, to 'suffer the slings and arrows' and walk proudly hand in hand with the person needing care. It puts a smile on your face. Both the care giver and the patient benefit, and life becomes worth living.

THIRTY-SEVEN

The Dementia Time Line for Deterioration

If I did not research evidence for what my wife, Marilyn, is going through, I would be remiss in doing all that is possible to understand the disease wiping away her mind and body. The Internet is a good source of material if you need to understand what is ahead for both patient and care giver. Under an article entitled, 'What is Psychology?', the stages of dementia leading to Alzheimer's is clearly spelled out, and seven stages are documented.

In stage 1, normal function is observed. No memory loss is recorded. In stage 2, very mild cognitive decline is evident. The patient may be concerned with mild symptoms of memory loss, but relatives and medical professionals can see no obvious symptoms of dementia during an exam or interview. In stage 3, things change. At this stage, mild cognitive decline is observed. Symptoms of Alzheimer's are now becoming obvious to other people in contact with the patient. Typical symptoms evident in stage 3 Alzheimer's include problems remembering names of people and objects, short-term memory issues and losing belongings, difficulties with organization and planning tasks or performing social or related tasks become more difficult. Stage 4 is a jump.

In stage 4, moderate cognitive decline is clearly evident. This is the first stage that is definitively classified as early-stage Alzheimer's. Symptoms detected will include short-term memory loss, problems performing complex tasks and challenging mental arithmetic, forgetfulness and changes in personality will come to the surface. At this stage, a decline of mental acuity is speeded up.

In stage 5, moderately severe cognitive decline evolves. This stage is classified as the mid-stage Alzheimer's and patients will show symptoms such as large gaps in memory and greater levels of confusion. The patient will also be less able to perform easier feats of mental arithmetic, but will still be capable of using the toilet and eating without assistance, although they might need help with some tasks.

In stage 6, there is severe cognitive decline, and it is this stage which is considered to be mid-range Alzheimer's. Patients will now need a great deal of help taking care of everyday tasks and memory problems will have worsened. Patients may have problems sleeping at night and lose control of their bladder and bowels. Behavior problems including paranoia and delusions might now be evident by this stage, and patients are likely to need constant supervision for their own safety.

Stage 7 introduces a very severe cognitive decline. This stage is classified as the late-stage Alzheimer's and it is the final stage of the disease. By now, the patient has lost the ability to respond their environment. They will require assistance with all aspects of their daily care and will probably be confined to bed. By the time a patient is in the final stage of Alzheimer's, the quality of life is greatly impaired. They often have difficulty swallowing and eating, and they are far more vulnerable to infection. This last stage can last for several years although many patients succumb to secondary infections quickly, and at this stage of the disease, the only real focus is to make the patient comfortable and treat them with as much passion and dignity as possible.

Marilyn, my wife of sixty-four years is somewhere between stages 4 and 5. I will do my very best to march in step right beside her on this hike through time. I have done thirty-mile marches in my life, but this is the most difficult forward effort I have ever made. But my hiking partner is not alone. Marilyn is the nicest person I have ever known. Her empathy for man and beast is second to none, and the prevailing winds are pushing us toward stages 6 and 7, a dangerous area full of the unknown. I do not look forward to such a place. But I will do everything possible to make transitions as pain-free as possible. Will I record that which is to come? Most likely. If along the way I learn of new and more-effective treatments and approaches, I will camp there and make them part of the arsenal in this unwinnable war. There will be no surrender here. I would like to look Dementia in the face and say, "I am your worst enemy; I am making my wife's trip as effortless as possible."

THIRTY-EIGHT

Advice and Consent

If I did not try to understand why people get dementia and Alzheimer's disease, I would be remiss in my effort to comprehend what my wife is experiencing. I did look into Alzheimer's Mayo Clinic report. It's title page began with 'Help Prevent Alzheimer's' and continued with 'Please donate.' That very tempting sale's pitch left me with a very bad taste in my mouth. So, I continued with a topic entitled, 'Are you having senior moments?'. That Internet article was written by a doctor who advocated dietary supplements as to how to avoid the disease. The physician cited the fact that one of three people will die of dementia in the U.S. The names of Charles Bronson, Rita Hayworth, Peter Falk and Perry Como were given as evidence that even celebrities die from the disease. I was still not impressed.

In the next section of the doctor's report, I was told that if your brain is getting the right nutrition and oxygen, then your brain remains healthy. 'Brain-friendly vitamins' were suggested, and the doctor's own, on-line remedy made with coconut oil was suggested, and for as little as $25.00, the first bottle would put you on the right track for brain recovery. Bovine scatology!

I have already cited the fact that over-the-counter medications do little to prevent or slow down the progression of the disease. And, in spite of the fact that I have never studied medicine, I do have some suggestions as to why Marilyn has lapsed into this awful slide toward an abyss. And, it must be remembered that this is a subjective opinion, but it costs nothing, and don't buy my book.

At the age of eighteen as a high-school graduate, Marilyn took a job by taking dictation in shorthand for a local county administrator. She worked at that job for a year before joining me overseas where I was deployed. After our return to the United States, she worked as a secretary at various offices and then took courses in ophthalmology and assisted ophthalmologists in several offices. And, then, after working long hours, Marilyn retired over twenty years ago, and stopped completely… no more mental stress or memorization of what should be done. She was at rest from the requirements of keeping up with the demands of the workplace. That mental inactivity contributed, I believe, to the onset of what is now dementia. I did just the opposite, and I hesitate to compare myself with Marilyn; she is so far above me I cannot even tie her shoes.

Years in the classroom, adding to my teaching credentials, traveling to three other countries to enhance skills, studying and trying to maintain the ability to speak French, Spanish and Japanese, picking up and studying how to play the banjo, guitar and harmonica and writing a few books has stimulated what few brain cells I had to begin with. In short, my advice to young adults would be this: do not stop learning. Make choices to enhance your knowledge of things which bring you happiness and pleasure. This advice might not work, but it will not cost you $25.00 a bottle. Now, I am going to make a healthy breakfast for Marilyn.

THIRTY-NINE

Faulty Diagnosis and Frustration

Thank goodness my doctorate is not in medicine. I am not sure I could handle more than one patient. Since Marilyn's hospital visit on December 17, for reasons of dizziness, she had been plagued with that symptom for over a week. That feature has manifested itself in the early hours of the morning after taking her medications. Such setbacks are recorded on her heart monitor, and I am sure that the message has been received. But I began to get curious, and I did some research on the Internet.

Marilyn is taking Amlodipine for blood pressure, Donepezil for dementia, Levothyroxine for hypothyroidism, Lisinopril for blood pressure and some over-the-counter vitamin supplements. Just for fun, I electronically inquired whether the above drugs would have an interaction. My findings were this: Amlodipine and Donepezil, taken together, do bring on drug interactions, and people who take both have interactions which cause tremors among females---characteristics of Marilyn's reaction. Dizziness, one of Marilyn's complaints, too, and this reaction is common when both drugs are taken together.

Marilyn's next appointment with her physician comes up early in January. Not soon enough. Starting tomorrow morning, Marilyn will not take Donepezil, her dementia pill, with other medications, something which might or might not stop the progression of the disease (results of tests are pending). Will I be scolded by Marilyn's physicians? Hell, I have been scolded by full-bird Marine Corps colonels. I thought it necessary to call the doctor's office today, and a message was left concerning my intended decisions. Even on weekends, some physicians return calls within twenty-four hours. As Marilyn's care giver, I made a decision. If I am right, and I think I am, I might write a book. Oh, and by the way, Marilyn took her first dose of coconut oil this afternoon…with yogurt. She wanted chocolate, but let's not stretch one's luck.

There is one more suggestion for the care giver in this situation regarding conscription medicine. Talk to your local pharmacist. Most often, they have a better understanding of drugs and their influence than the physician. I will follow up with our pharmacists today.

FORTY

The Spirit of the Season and a Turn for the Better

It, this turn for the good, is beyond my comprehension. Whether it was the coconut oil, the timing of when certain medications are taken with each other, or last evening's sitting out at the bar on our patio with Christmas lights burning brightly, something better has taken place. For the first time in a month, Marilyn's blood pressure count, 114/55, was back to normal.

Yesterday at the pharmacy, in consultation with a young male pharmacist, it was agreed that dispensation of certain medicines would take place at different times during the day. As, usual, I was wearing some Marine Corps clothing, and before I left the pharmacy, my pharmacist said, "Semper Fi! I was with the 2-12 in Afghanistan." Everyone seems to be helping lately. Advice on things such as coconut supplements, pill taking, heart monitoring and casual get togethers add to the mix of things for the better. Could be the season, too.

Last evening for the first time this winter, temperatures allowed Marilyn and I to sit out on our patio. I made sure Marilyn dressed warmly in spite of the mid-60's mercury reading, and we enjoyed our well-lit Christmas-like lights. Passers-by said hello, we exchanged both Christmas and Hanukkah greetings and enjoyed handing out treats to the neighbors' dogs. I look forward to a repeat of last evening's outing. No tremors, no dizziness, and I felt myself in the right place at the right time with the right person. I might give in to Marilyn's request that she take her medications with chocolate instead of with yogurt. Addictions are a terrible thing to control. After all, I am Marilyn's care giver.

FORTY-ONE

The Repetition of Questions

From what I have observed with Marilyn, the dementia patient's mind does hold on to recent events and seeks answers to what might seem like a threat. In our area, still not quite tamed, we have coyotes, rattle snakes and javelina seen regularly. The coyotes are nocturnal, and are rarely seen. However, if pet dogs are let out at night without their owner, the dogs disappear. Our rattle snakes are mostly found several miles away in the mountains, and as of this time, none have been seen in our gated community. That cannot be said about our javelinas.

I use the possessive pronoun, 'ours' because the javelina are native to our region. They were here before us, and they are still here. Their diet consists of decorative Southwestern plants which surround our compound. The name peccary is sometimes used to describe the animal, and, for the most part, they are not dangerous unless accompanied by their young. It is not a good idea to pet them. Some of our residents want them destroyed, but I am among those who say, let them be. They add color. But not to Marilyn.

Marilyn loves animals, but she also respects them. This morning, on one of her short walks, one of our residents, a man, (she has no idea who) drove up to her and asked that Marilyn retrace her steps. Not far away was one of the bigger javelina taking his morning stroll. The automobile driver backed his car and waited until Marilyn was in her condo. Nice gesture on the part of one of our residents.

Marilyn came in our unit, related the story to me and asked, "If I see one of those animals again, what do I do?" I was tempted to say to Marilyn, 'What you don't do is walk up to the animal and say', "Here kitty, kitty". So, I told my wife that the good Samaritan had done the right thing; he had led her away from possible danger. That same question has been repeated four times today. Such repetitiveness must not be misinterpreted. It is part of the dementia patient's trying to make sense of a new and different world. I held off the 'Here, kitty, kitty' suggestion. By this evening, that mental picture of the javelina will have been washed away with the Sun's disappearance over the horizon. And, then the coyotes come out. We don't have a dog.

FORTY-TWO

Fainting Spells and Last-Minute Advice

This morning, after our ritual of taking medications, recording blood pressure and having coffee, Marilyn lost consciousness, and I caught her before she hit the floor. That experience was recorded electronically and forwarded to our physician with whom we have a follow-up appointment in early January. She was nauseous and needed to do a bowel movement. Nothing will be related about that other than saying that the care giver has many responsibilities during the day and should be aware that attention is often needed. Marilyn is resting now, and I will check on her often. There will be no pickle ball this morning.

As for those who in the future will find themselves playing the role of the care giver to a dementia/Alzheimer's patient, let me reiterate and embellish on some of the things I have learned. First of all, you might not be able to choose your patient. If the afflicted person is a spouse, relative or immediate family member, the things which bind you to that person will dictate the approach you take in performing your role. In my case, I was lucky; my patient is my wife, the woman I have loved for many years. Such an attachment makes my job easier, and I would not want to give up my place to another. Little things will come to mind. You might have to give up playing golf or some other sport such as pickle ball. Unless you are a national champion at a sport, no one is going to miss you on the links or on the courts. Use the time you spent hitting a ball to perfect your new game, that of offering personal care to someone who needs you.

You, the care giver, are most likely not a person with a medical degree. Medications and their dispensation will become confusing. Wrong dosages will cause flareups of all sorts of symptoms with the patient. Be calm, make arrangements to remedy the wrong and go on with your care. Your patient will lose her appetite. You will blame yourself for your ineptitude. Don't! You have no control over the mind and body of your patient. The patient's mind doesn't either. But there is more.

The care giver will find that he or she is not alone. Friends of both the care giver and the patient will offer advice. Quite often, they, these kind-hearted people, have experienced the disease up close or they know someone who has. These people are great sources of information. Listen to them. If you are able, do your own research. Your physician is very busy with multiple patients and will not be aware of all you have experienced. Use discretion, but be ready to use common sense. You know your patient better than most professionals, and you must be ready to make decisions. Remain calm; your patient reacts to emotion. Present a solid front, stand firm and be tolerant. Win the battle.

FORTY-THREE

The Transition from the Familiar to the Unfamiliar

Dr. Allen R. Remaley

Marilyn grew up in the coal fields of Western Pennsylvania. Her father was a clay and coal miner. In her home, hand pumps supplied water from a local spring to the home. Indoor plumbing was outside…in a two-hole. Marilyn helped her mother with household chores, attended church with her family and was usually the last after her older brothers to use the bath water in a wash tub twice a week. In her younger days, electronic appliances were scarce. Not so much now, but still things have changed.

During her married life, Marilyn did have electronic appliances such as a washer and dryer. She had used them well, and always made sure that sheets, pillow cases and clothing were properly cleaned. However, now, dementia has erased knowledge of the use of the once easily manipulated dials and levers of operation of most machines. This morning, always ready to help around the home, Marilyn called to me and asked for help. She had loaded the washer with clothing ready to be washed and wanted me to check. We found that laundry soap had not been added first---a qualification with our machine. We emptied the wash tub, added laundry detergent and once again added the dirty clothes. But we had some new learning to take place.

Although she had been shown how to set the dials on the washer and begin the process several times before, a new learning was required. I wondered whether my teaching skills had dwindled. A lot of my former students probably questioned that, too. But I knew that things already covered needed tweaking. There is nothing wrong with a re-play of learning, and it is the care giver who does the reteaching and thus preserving the dignity of the dementia patient. And, it doesn't end there. After the clothes cycle has ended, the same application of learning must take place with the dryer. Once I have finished my lesson on both the washer and dryer…for the day, I say to my wife, "You know, Hon. These new-fangled washing machines confuse me, too. I think Elon Musk invented them." I love laundry day.

FORTY-FOUR

The Wonderful Gift of Slumber

Lately, Marilyn is again exhibiting something unusual. She is taking naps. For her, as long as I have known her, she has always been on the move, actively engaged in either work around the home and hands-on projects. But now, Marilyn has become attached to her new 'My Pillow', a well-promoted item to the American public. She has also become an aficionado of my recliner, the thing on which I have slept for the last fifteen years.

At first, I thought that her inclination to catch a few winks was her approval of my study of Spanish and that a siesta would fit in the scheme of things. As you might expect, I did some research on the Mayo Clinic website, and information tells me that a person suffering from dementia does spend time sleeping, and that rest is both soothing and eliminates stressful moments. I now must wonder whether dementia is contagious. I, too, slip into that silent pathway to dreams from time to time. Sleep well, my dear. It's OK.

FORTY-FIVE

Recess and the Care Giver

There will come times when the care giver becomes tired, begins to question his or her own actions or efficiency, and senses the stress of the moment creeping into the subconscious. The tasks of the job, reteaching, coaching, observing, clearing up misconceptions, meal preparation…all sorts of things, will sometimes drain strength and enthusiasm needed by the care giver. Be careful! Stress and confusion are not restricted to the dementia patient. You, the care giver, might need a break.

No, don't rush out and book a flight to the beaches of Hawaii. They are now populated by scores of homeless. Don't jump on the first plane to a Club Med village. But a pause in the action might be called for to recharge your battery. Our new electric automobiles can travel hundreds of miles, but eventually, they, too, need recharging. Before you go flying off to a place of relaxation, make sure that your patient is safe and well-cared for.

You will not always find a kind person to relieve you from your duties. Make sure that your patient is in a place where he can function without your presence for a time to be determined only by you. No one knows your patient better than you. If you do need to leave your station for an hour or more, determine whether your patient can be on his own for any duration of time. My patient, Marilyn, does want to know where I am going. If I need to get groceries, pick up prescriptions, etc., I give a time for my return. I might stop for a cup of coffee, make a side-bar stop for ice cream for both of us, but those short outings are usually enough for me to reboot. And, the care giver's short absence might even be to the advantage of the patient. None of us are that good.

FORTY-SIX

Closure

I don't like the word. It signals termination. But Marilyn and I are closing in on the beginning of stage six in a seven-stage explanation of where dementia sweeps up an innocent victim and deposits the remains. In earlier writings, the symptoms of each of the seven stages of the disease were outlined. I am reluctant to reveal such development to friends and supporters. Such things should remain exclusive to the care giver. Instead, let me share some of the every-day expressions of appreciation from the woman who knows what is ailing her but does not understand why.

Marilyn will often say, "I am so blessed." She is aware that she is not alone. Often heard is, "How can I help you?" She is always ready to lend a hand if needed. "What can I get for you?" is heard. When asked, "Marilyn, would you be so kind as to set the table for us?", some of the requested items will be missing. If I have to eat off the end of a knife, I will do so. Leif Ericson did. Doesn't work so well with peas, but we rarely have them.

This afternoon when I go over to the community room to set up for tomorrow's New Year's Eve get together, a shadow will follow me and ask, "How can I help?" Marilyn will be there right beside me. Fireworks? Not so much. But one thing is sure. I will have the perfect partner for New Year's Eve…and beyond. Happy New Year, folks.

FORTY-SEVEN

The Train

Recently, the trip we take through life was equated with that of a train ride. Our ticket is stamped at birth, and we travel through many places. Stops are made along the way. Some people get off, some get on and the clackety-clack of the train's wheels sometimes puts us to sleep. Along the way, we meet some interesting fellow travelers. We acknowledge them, converse with them and share our stories. Some of the riders meet, fall in love with and marry along the way, perhaps at one of the scheduled stops.

Big cities, vast forests, vacation spots, churches, cathedrals and synagogues can be seen outside as the train passes by. Wonderful sights and passengers will be heard saying, "Did you see that? What a great show nature is putting on!" Marilyn's train is picking up speed every day, and it is racing toward an unknown destination. She is not alone.

During the past weeks and months, I have made an effort to describe what might be required of a care giver to a dementia patient. This guide is by no means the definitive edition of what steps one should take in preserving the dignity and passion of the person afflicted with the disease. Each dementia patient is different, and they require their own map which will help them along the way. Others are, at this moment, working up their own GPS document hoping that their own guide works well for both patient and care giver. As for me, I am having the ride of my life, and I am not alone.

FORTY-EIGHT

Cloaking

It was my intention to close this manuscript and stop documenting my wife's struggle with the disease. But there are too many discoveries that occur each day, and my comprehension of them is not clear. This morning, after our ritual of coffee, news updates, pill taking, blood pressure recording and hydration, we began our writing. Each day we sit opposite each other and put down what to expect during the day. After a few minutes, the only thing on Marilyn's paper was, 'Monday, January 2, 2023'.

I spoke to Marilyn and assured her that the number of words on a paper is not the important matter. I then made breakfast. Marilyn could not eat her food. She started to cry and said, "I don't know what's happening to me. I just don't know…" After a warm and hopefully comforting hug, I escorted Marilyn to her bedroom and made sure that she was warm and at peace. Once that was done, I closed her bedroom door and tried to analyze what had just occurred. I failed.

Within the past few days, I have noticed something else. The things we see clearly, those various everyday objects with which we have become familiar, become invisible to the dementia patient. Such things as a plastic measuring cup, once manipulated with culinary skill, becomes cloaked by the mind's vocabulary, and if the thing observed cannot be described, it is concealed as if covered by a blanket. Marilyn is at rest now. She is not alone. God is with her. So am I.

FORTY-NINE

Recapitulation

At the end of some Hollywood films, some of the more important scenes are shown to the audience. Sometimes, just to aid memory, the subject of this manuscript, a review of things discussed does help. We already know that dementia/Alzheimer's offers no cure. Yes, institutions such as the American Alzheimer's Association and the Mayo Clinic are conducting experiments, but there is yet no light at the end of the tunnel. Dementia is very much like an avalanche. It comes roaring down the mountain side with such force that no earthly means can stop its surge to the bottom. But those who survive the onslaught, deserve care. And that is the job of the care giver.

Dementia's warning signs need to be observed. Disruptions in daily living. Changes in temperament, eating habits, the misplacement of personal property and associations with others need to be observed. Should warning signs warrant professional opinion, appointments must be made and testing carried out. Should a diagnosis point toward the beginning of the disease, other things must be followed up.

Special diets might be called for, hydration should be monitored, and arrangements for the patient's association with others should be considered. Daily routines, the norm, should be emphasized and practiced. But the number one rule of thumb is this: preserve the dignity and humanity of the patient. Ease them toward the finality of life. It's the one thing which will give both the patient and the care giver a reason for being.

Addendum: Yesterday, December 6, 2023, the FDA granted accelerated approval of lecanemab, marketed under the name of Lequembi. In trials, the drug showed promise for slowing the cognitive decline in early and mild Alzheimer's disease. However, swelling and bleeding in the brain is possible. The cost of the drug, $26,000 a year is also a problem for most people.

There is yet one weapon to use against a brain which continues to distort the reality of the memory of your dementia patient. Sometimes, the patient is unaware of the power of positive thinking and free will. Recently, our son, Brooks, sent a box of Electrolit to his mother. The flavored liquid is used to rehydrate those who are in need of fluids in their body. Marilyn has been drinking the foreign-made beverage for weeks, and whether or not that extra hydration is having an effect or not, Marilyn's awareness of her surroundings has improved.

I spoke to Marilyn this morning saying, "Hon, I think that the liquid you are drinking has a lot to do with what seems to be an improvement in how you are doing from day to day." Marilyn's eyes lit up, and she said, "Do you think so?" Of course, I agreed. Using reverse psychology on the dementia patient's mind, i.e., having her believe that the things she does has a positive effect on her life, could be another weapon in our arsenal against the disease. After all, the brain is conducting its own war and is sometimes unaware of the patient's will to live.

FIFTY

The Choices We Make

Dr. Allen R. Remaley

In the late 40's and 50's, the institution which takes in abandoned children, Boy's Town, used a logo which pictured a young boy carrying a smaller child on his back. The boy carrying the other was looking up at a clergyman, and the caption read, "He ain't heavy, Father. He's my brother." The humanity expressed in that picture has stuck with me over all these years, and this morning's pickle ball outing brought back the reality of being a care giver to a dementia patient.

My wife and I try to play pickle ball at least three times a week, and we are on the courts by 8 A.M. This morning, however, there was a problem. Marilyn, still in her pajamas, said to me, "I have nothing to wear." What she was really telling me was, 'I am having trouble dressing myself this morning.' In our little vacation home, we have several clothes closets. I have been allocated a two by three-foot section of one of those closets. In all the other ones, there are dresses, skirts, pull-overs, sweat pants and shirts, sweaters and shoes. All of those items sport designs of floral arrangements, pictures of bunnies, butterflies and hearts. There is no lack of feminine wear in our home. Marilyn and I looked through some of the clothes on display, and for the first time in memory, I helped dress Marilyn for an outing. But you know, folks, she ain't heavy. She's my wife.

FIFTY-ONE

The Secretary/Record Keeper

Not to be overlooked, if you become a care giver for a dementia patient, is the fact that tabulation of certain necessary things must take place. There are times when I feel that I am in the movie, 'Groundhog Day' and that I am repeating my freshman year in college; there are so many new things to keep in mind. Marilyn's blood pressure has been high, and an effort to regulate it has taken place. According to physicians and pharmacists, blood pressure drugs should be taken at night before bedtime. Some of these medicines cause dizziness, and it is better that the patient be in bed should that happen.

Blood pressure readings are taken in the morning, body temperature is recorded and hydration fluids and their ingestion are monitored. I am now becoming more aware of what Lisinopril, Donepezil, Amlodipine and Levothyroxine do. No, you will not earn a doctorate in chemistry, but you will be more knowledgeable about the drugs and become sensitive to what might be drug interactions.

The dementia patient should in no way be made responsible for record keeping, times of drug administering or schedules. That causes stress. Do keep in mind that the care giver is not immune to such things either. However, the satisfaction of seeing that positive results come from appropriate care will be rewarding.

FIFTY-TWO

The Sound of Music

Another observation/recommendation to my fellow care givers is this. Determine whether or not music, tunes which might have once been familiar to your dementia patient, plays a part in brightening the day. Whether it be CD's, radio, the Music Channel on TV or something you, the care giver, devise, if familiar sounds open the door to cognitive sensitivity, use that tool. You, yourself, might even enjoy it.

For some reason, about thirteen years ago, I purchased a used banjo, began to take lessons and, after a few years, I could play 'Dueling Banjos' and other well-known five-string banjo tunes. Marilyn, always ready to compliment me on my efforts, got into the habit of sitting near me when I play. Lately, I invested in a cheap guitar, and skills built up in my banjo playing transferred automatically to my other five-string instrument.

I have been polishing my renditions of Blake Shelton's, 'Old Red', Toby Keith's, 'I love this bar', and Chris Jansen's, 'Buy me a boat'. Marilyn takes a seat near me, overlooks my mistakes in music theory and smiles her kind approval of my playing. The smile on her face says it all. She is made aware that her care giver is doing something just for her, and her smile is transferred to me.

Am I advocating that every dementia care giver become a musician? Not hardly. Everyone has some little skill, trick or talent. Find out what it is, practice it, determine whether it has a positive effect on your patient...and use it as part of your arsenal in this battle against the most insidious of enemies. If whatever you do to entertain and make lighter the burden of your dementia patient works, you have come away a winner.

Friday morning, I invested in a Home Mini music player. I ordered in in the morning. It arrived from Amazon this afternoon. The music emitted from the little, round music box is good. But Marilyn still enjoys my string instruments. Having a back up helps.

FIFTY-THREE

The Patient and Patience

Every day, I learn something new about being a care giver. My wife is teaching me self-restraint. In her state, she is not quick to interpret distance and positioning of objects. If, for example, I am busy with other things (preparing meals, counting out medications, or doing what should be done during the day), and the phone rings, I might say, "Hon, the phone is ringing, and it is near the sink. Could you get it?" In that one verbal expression of need, there are several entities which come into play, and they all require cognitive action. The phone, something once automatic in its manipulation, might now be foreign. Its sound, once so clearly recognizable and easily located, is now challenging. The sink, an object easily located in the past, might now be unfamiliar and not often used. The care giver must be aware of these subtle changes.

There is no cause for alarm in missing a phone call. If important, the caller will make an effort to reach you later. Hesitancy of response must be understood and tolerated. At some stage in our lives, we will learn that time, if we take it seriously and know that we have a lot of it, especially those of us who have left our careers behind, will allow for tolerance and understanding. Use patience with your dementia patient. Both patient and care giver will benefit.

FIFTY-FOUR

A Box of Chocolates

When Forest Gump uttered his famous, "Life is like a box of chocolates; you never know what you're going to get.", little did I know that his phrase would become appropriate in my association as a dementia care giver. In our condo building, friends get together every evening about 5 P.M. and talk about the day's events. Before that gathering, I had involved Marilyn in my latest pastime---guitar playing and adapting some country/western lyrics to music. We had been working on Chris Jansen's, 'It could buy me a boat'. In that song, a redneck story teller speaks of his not having enough money to buy a boat. Working with Marilyn, I would voice a few lines having to do with situations which might allow the redneck come up with enough money for his purchase.

In last night's get together, about a dozen people sat around our tables and showed cell phone pictures of family and past outings. One of our participants was passing around his automobile repair bill he had just received. Doug, the car owner, has a high-end automobile, and his repair bill matches in price and then some. Marilyn was sitting next to Doug, and she became interested in what he was saying. At that point, I interrupted to conversations and asked for one minute's attention while Marilyn and I gave a rendition of our gig which would take us to Vegas.

I got out my guitar, asked Marilyn is she was ready, and I gave the first few bars and lyrics to the song. At a well-practiced point, Marilyn was supposed to chime in, "It could buy me a boat." Remember the repair bill? When it came time for Marilyn's one-liner, she sang out,

"It could buy me a car." Almost immediately, Marilyn realized that she had picked the wrong piece of chocolate. Almost in tears, and now realizing her faux pas, Marilyn apologized for her misstep. I gave her a hug and said, "Hon, no one here knows the lyrics to the song. We might even change the wording. Besides, there are no ocean-front properties in Arizona." Ah, the surprises in store for a dementia care giver. May they keep coming.

FIFTY-FIVE

Final Message

What might be some of the last pieces of advice that I feel should be given to a dementia care giver? Let me begin by saying that there is no sure panacea for the mental anguish, depression or the sense of frustration you will encounter. You are not God. There is no remedy for all of life's illnesses. But you, the care giver, are in control. Knowing that, realizing that you are the pilot, the wheelman, the driver of whatever vehicle you imagine, make plans to do well. Build humor and frivolity into your trip. Smiles come from and go immediately into the brain, and they act as a balm which sooths. Know, too, that you need to take time to recharge the batteries which power your machine. Make it, this trip you will take, be a good one. Make good memories happen. There will come a time when you need them. Oh, one more thing. Your dementia patient will never be like Marilyn.

FIFTY-SIX

Nice Patients and Mean Patients

One last but important item should be expressed to a potential dementia-care giver. Last evening at our January's special event, 'Crock-Pot Night', over a dozen attendees dined on various preparations and enjoyed the evening together. During our get together, one of the guests came up to me and asked, "How's Marilyn doing?" Without hesitation, I responded, "Marilyn is doing super well. She is upbeat and smiling. She's a treasure." My interlocutor answered, "You are lucky. You have a 'nice' Marilyn. My aunt had a 'mean' Marilyn." I asked my fellow 'crock-pot' devotee to explain, and he told me that sometimes, the dementia patient can be nasty, uncooperative and reluctant to accept direction. I understood.

If a care giver is saddled with such an unpleasant patient, someone who during his life did not respect ethnic, social or religious differences, the care giver must immediately devise a battle plan, a plan of action which will preserve the dignity and passion of both the care giver and patient. Designing such a plan will take time, and professional advice should be sought. Once the plan is firmly established, it must be put into action.

In my case, my 'nice' Marilyn was raised in a family whose members believed in God. They believed that kindness would override evil, and that patience was golden. The care giver who does not give in to belligerence will feel better and benefit. And, that 'mean' patient's reluctancy might be displaced by what one man once said: "Forgive them, Father, for they know not what they do."

Fin

ACKNOWLEDGEMENTS

For some time, Marilyn's friends and acquaintances have expressed their support and best wishes. I will have missed some of those kind people because of my own lack of memory.

Fran Riggs, Ed Heyen, Douglas Graham, Greg Patrei, Jean Wacker, Cami Wacker, Marcus Wacker, Dave Ross, Mike Salisbury, Barbara Landis, Mary Ann Villala, Chana Anderson, Sara Abraham Wood, Judith Lebeaux Aleksa, Roger Aleksa, Susan Williams, Diana Bustillo De Ohmstedt, Colleen OConner Potter, Shelly Hiemestra, Randy Grimm, Rebecca Brynteson Conner, Carol Pletz, Blasé Iuliano, Carol Snyder Valdez, Joann Allender, Robert Allender, Deanna Baughman, Rex Baughman, Roger Baughman, Gloria Baughman, Galen Baughman, Grace Landes, Jeff Vredenberg, Brenda Vredenberg, Jude Weisand, E. Foulk, Joyce Foulk, Cathy Pallman, Douglas Pallman, Dave Carpenter, Denise Carpenter, Walt Tapper, Alice Tapper, John Cherveny, Irene Cherveny, Charlene Prince, Mike Decker, Michelle Decker, Janine Remaley Hawthorne, Brooks M. Remaley, Janis Margaret Haggard, Douglas Mills, Bob Landis, Carol Van Dyke, Marty Van Dyke,